Practical Hysteroscopy

Practical Hysteroscopy

PATRICK J. TAYLOR MD, FRCS(C), FRCOG
Chairman of Department of Obstetrics & Gynaecology,
St Paul's Hospital, Vancouver,
and Professor of Obstetrics & Gynaecology,
University of British Columbia,
Vancouver, Canada

AND

ALAN G. GORDON FRCS, FRCOG
Honorary Consultant Gynaecologist,
Princess Royal Hospital, Hull, UK

FOREWORD BY
CARL J. LEVINSON MD

OXFORD
Blackwell Scientific Publications
LONDON EDINBURGH BOSTON
MELBOURNE PARIS BERLIN VIENNA

© 1993 by
Blackwell Scientific Publications
Editorial Offices:
Osney Mead, Oxford OX2 0EL
25 John Street, London WC1N 2BL
23 Ainslie Place, Edinburgh EH3 6AJ
238 Main Street, Cambridge
 Massachusetts 02142, USA
54 University Street, Carlton
 Victoria 3053, Australia

Other Editorial Offices:
Librairie Arnette SA
2, rue Casimir-Delavigne
75006 Paris
France

Blackwell Wissenschafts-Verlag GmbH
Düsseldorfer Str. 38
D-10707 Berlin
Germany

Blackwell MZV
Feldgasse 13
A-1238 Wien
Austria

First published 1993

Set by Semantic Graphics Services,
Singapore
Printed and bound in Great Britain
at the University Press, Cambridge

DISTRIBUTORS

Marston Book Services Ltd
PO Box 87, Oxford OX2 0DT
(*Orders*: Tel: 0865 791155
        Fax: 0865 791927
        Telex: 837515)

USA
Blackwell Scientific Publications, Inc.
238 Main Street
Cambridge, MA 02142
(*Orders*: Tel: 800 759–6102
           617 876–7000)

Canada
Times Mirror Professional
Publishing, Ltd, 130 Flaska Drive
Markham, Ontario L6G 1B8
(*Orders*: Tel: 800 268–4178
           416 470–6739)

Australia
Blackwell Scientific Publications
Pty Ltd, 54 University Street
Carlton, Victoria 3053
(*Orders*: Tel: 03 347–5552)

A catalogue record for this title
is available from the British Library

ISBN 0-632-03672-9

Library of Congress
Cataloging-in-Publication Data

Taylor, Patrick J.
  Practical hysteroscopy/
Patrick J. Taylor and Alan G. Gordon.
     p.   cm.
  Companion vol. to: Practical
laparoscopy/Alan G. Gordon and
Patrick J. Taylor.
  Includes bibliographical references
and index.
  ISBN 0-632-03672-9
  1. Uterus—Endoscopic surgery.
  2. Hysteroscopy. I. Gordon, Alan G.
II. Gordon, Alan G. Practical
laparoscopy.   III. Title.
  [DNLM:1. Genital Diseases, Female—
diagnosis.
  2. Genital Diseases. Female—surgery.
  3. Hysteroscopy—methods.
WP 141 T245p]
RG104.7.T39   1993
618.1'45—dc20
DNML/DLC
for Library of Congress

Contents

Foreword

CARL J. LEVINSON*

'Wisdom is meaningless unless your experience has given it meaning
... and there is wisdom in the selection of wisdom.' [Bergan Evans]

Although the concept of hysteroscopy is two centuries old, the
practical aspects have only begun to emerge in the last two decades.
Modern technology has transformed what was a difficult diagnostic
procedure into remarkable diagnostic access to the intra-uterine
cavity with capability for operative intervention where indicated. In
essence, therapy may be instituted at the same time as diagnosis is
made.

This practical manual fulfills its commitment to the reader. Once
the principles have been established the reader is led carefully from
instrumentation to diagnostic hysteroscopy with caveats regarding
pre-operative investigation. Once comfortable in this arena, it is a
natural step forward to simple operations followed, with experience,
by more complex operative procedures. Training begets safety and
safety begets avoidance of complications but the authors have been
clear as to how complications can be managed, should they occur.

The authors are experienced and bring together both British and
North American concepts on the subject. The reader will be de-
lighted by the clarity of presentation and the vivid delineation of
subject. The book serves well as a 'quick refresher' but also as a
comprehensive review of the subject of hysteroscopy.

This manual presents its subject with comprehension, practicality,
surgical expertise and refined medical behavior ... as is befitting the
competence of the authors.

'The best effect of any book is that it excites the reader to self
activity.' [Thomas Carlyle]

* Director, Stanford Endoscopy Center for Training & Technology, and Associate
Professor, Department of Gynecology & Obstetrics, Stanford University School of
Medicine, San Francisco, USA.

Preface

Until recently hysteroscopy was used by a few enthusiasts primarily as a diagnostic procedure. The last few years have seen enormous advances in our ability to carry out advanced hysteroscopic surgery. Few can argue with the advantages of this approach. The saving to patients both from discomfort and in the time necessary for hospitalization and return to normal function is enormous. Fiscal advantages accrue to those who must pay for health care. Many of these procedures have been developed since practising gynaecologists finished their training. Endoscopic surgery should now be an integral part of the experience of junior staff.

This book and its companion *Practical Laparoscopy* have been written to serve as guides for clinicians who wish to develop additional endoscopic skills. It is hoped that they will provide solid didactic foundations for those undertaking such further training.

P.J.T., A.G.G.

Acknowledgements

The authors wish to express their appreciation for technical assistance to the following companies: ICI Pharmaceuticals (UK), Wilmslow, Cheshire, UK, and Karl Storz GmbH, Mittelstrasse 8, 7200 Tuttlingen, Germany.

1: Introduction

Modern endoscopy has advanced since Bozzini in 1805 peered into the urethra of a living subject and, for his pains, was promptly censured by the Medical Faculty at the University of Vienna for 'undue curiosity'. Curiosity, not necessity, has been the true mother of invention. This 'how to' book could not have been written if physicians and scientists had not kept asking 'what if?'

The answers to the questions have arrived with amazing rapidity. The 'what if we put a telescope into the uterine cavity?' was followed by 'what if we distended the cavity with gas or fluid?'

The early telescopes were of large diameter and had inferior systems for illumination. 'What if we improved the lens system, and transmitted light through fibre-optic cable from an external source?' was answered by the engineers who have developed the cold light source and modern endoscopic equipment, of which the panoramic hysteroscope is a fine example. But diagnostic hysteroscopists were not long satisfied.

Could we add a system of magnifying lenses? The result was the invention of the microcolpohysteroscope, an instrument with which cellular observations can be made *in vivo*.

The truly curious have an overwhelming desire to tinker. Observing simply was not good enough. Would it be possible, after all our colleagues in urology work in a similar environment, to operate in the uterus? Addition of laser and electrosurgical equipment to the hysteroscope has answered this final question with a very definite affirmative. To all of this hysteroscopic equipment has been added the refinement of the silicone chip video camera, which permits diagnostic and operative procedures to be displayed on a video monitor. We remember Bozzini. The names of his less curious contemporaries are long forgotten.

Curiosity is also the reason that gynaecologists wish to improve their diagnostic and therapeutic skills. It is hoped that this book will in some part serve to satisfy and to stimulate that curiosity.

A number of excellent scholarly texts are available. The purpose of this book is to provide clear, unambiguous information about the capabilities of modern hysteroscopy.

The instruments will be described in detail. Once familiar with the equipment, the next logical step is to carry out diagnostic procedures. These will be discussed. Perhaps the most exciting advance in the field is the ability to perform both minor and more complex operative procedures by hysteroscopic means. The pre-operative investigation and management will be discussed in general terms. A step by step description of the minor procedures will be followed by a similar approach to the more complex. The indications, contra-indications, complications and their management and prevention will be discussed fully.

The book concludes with consideration of safety and training of the hysteroscopist. While curiosity has been lauded, its effects upon the cat must not be forgotten. No one should embark upon a new surgical approach until they are trained and comfortable with both the technique and the management of any complications which may arise.

It is to be hoped that the reader will find in these pages a comprehensive guide to the safe and very satisfying performance of both diagnostic and operative hysteroscopy.

2: Instruments

Introduction

The uterus has a potential cavity. To perform hysteroscopy accurately the cavity must be distended. The hysteroscope itself is a telescope which may provide varying degrees of magnification. The telescope can be fitted into a variety of external sheaths all of which serve the primary function of carrying the distension medium. Those sheaths used for purely diagnostic purposes serve no other function. If operative procedures are to be performed, sheaths have been designed either with channels through which ancillary instruments, including laser-bearing fibres, can be passed, or with instruments which are integral to the sheath. The simplest of these latter is equipped with scissors. The most complex and versatile instrument is a modification of the urological resectoscope. Illumination is provided by a cold light source and transmitted through fibre-optic or fluid-filled cables. Energy sources required for operative procedures include electrosurgical generators and lasers. The findings can be recorded using line drawings, still cameras or video recorders.

Distension media and their methods of delivery

The uterus may be distended with:
1 carbon dioxide;
2 a variety of fluids including:
  (a) saline;
  (b) dextrose;

(c) high molecular weight dextran;
(d) sorbitol;
(e) glycine.

Carbon dioxide

Carbon dioxide is the medium which gives the clearest view and is ideal for diagnostic purposes. It can only be used with the smaller telescopes. It is unsuitable for all but the simplest operative procedures because if there is any bleeding the resultant bubbles obliterate the view. Smoke generated if laser or electrosurgical energies are used with carbon dioxide also obscures the field of vision. Only equipment designed specifically for hysteroscopy can be used to deliver carbon dioxide. Most insufflators are either fixed flow/variable pressure or fixed pressure/variable flow. The micro-hysteroflator controls both the flow rate and the pressure. To ensure safety the rate of flow should not exceed 100 ml/minute and the pressure should remain below an absolute maximum of 200 mmHg (Fig. 2.1).

Liquid distension media

There is no perfect liquid distension medium. The advantages and disadvantages of each will be described. All, with the exception of high molecular weight dextran, can be delivered with an automatic pump or simply from the bag, either by gravity feed or by wrapping the bag in a blood pressure cuff which is inflated to a pressure

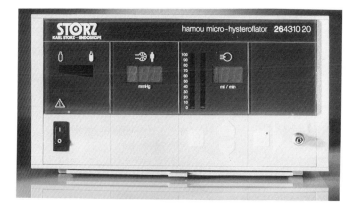

Fig. 2.1 Automatic gas insufflator for hysteroscopy.

between 80 and 100 mmHg. The pump which is marketed as the Hysteromat, like the hysteroflator, automatically controls the rate of flow and pressure (Fig. 2.2). As intravasation of fluid is an ever present risk, the automatic pump provides a greater margin of safety. In either case the bag or pump are connected to the inflow stopcock of the sheath by means of plastic tubing. High molecular weight dextran is too viscous to be instilled by gravity, is not produced in bags, and tends to clog the pump. It must be instilled from a 20–50 cc syringe.

Saline

Normal saline is isotonic, thus carrying no risk of haemolysis if intravasation occurs. It is cheap and readily available. Laser energy can be transmitted through saline but because of its electrolyte content it is dangerous if used with electrosurgical equipment. Current can be transmitted through the fluid and cause burns to intra-abdominal organs. It is miscible with blood, thus the field of vision becomes obscured if bleeding occurs.

Dextrose

Dextrose 5% in water is isotonic, miscible with blood, and if intravasation occurs, may cause hyperglycaemia. It is cheap and readily available.

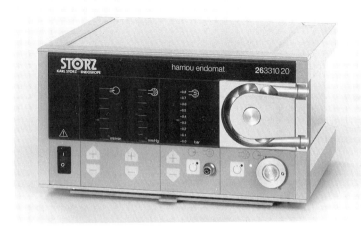

Fig. 2.2 Automatic fluid pump for hysteroscopic surgery.

Sorbitol

Sorbitol is a 3% solution of D-glucitol. It is an excellent medium for use with electrosurgical equipment. It is miscible with blood, and slightly hypotonic. If absorbed in large quantities, haemolysis may occur. Diabetics are at risk of hyperglycaemia.

Glycine

Glycine is an amino acid in 1.5% solution. It is non-haemolytic and is an excellent medium for use with electrical equipment. Intravasation may result in nausea, vertigo and high output cardiac failure. Its metabolites may produce encephalopathy if there is excessive intravasation of the solution.

High molecular weight dextran ('Hyskon')

Hyskon is a solution of 32% dextran. It is extremely viscous. It is only very slightly miscible with blood, but will not flow rapidly enough if irrigation is required to flush debris. It caramelizes on electrosurgical electrodes and can jam the working parts of pumps and hysteroscopic sheaths. It is a very useful medium for simple, non-bloody procedures. Intravasation may cause anaphylaxis or pulmonary oedema.

Telescopes

Conventional hysteroscopes, which are modified cystoscopes, and the microcolpohysteroscope are used in daily practice.

Conventional hysteroscopes

Most telescopes are conventional rigid optical instruments with a proximal eyepiece and a distal lens which may have an angle of 0 or 30°. The former permits direct visualization, the latter a fore-oblique view. They range in diameter from 3.5 to 6 mm. A flexible telescope with a steerable tip is available.

The microcolpohysteroscope

The Hamou 1 instrument (Karl Storz GmbH & Co., Tuttlingen, Germany) is a complex optical system which possesses the properties of both the telescope and the compound microscope (Fig. 2.3). It can

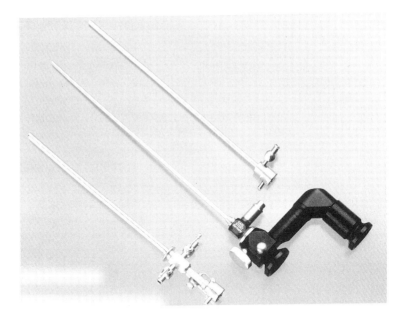

Fig. 2.3 Hamou 1 microcolpohysteroscope.

be used at infinity as a telescope, or in contact with the epithelium as a microscope. The telescope is 4 mm in diameter and 25 cm in length. There are two proximal lenses, the direct lens allows observation at unity, the conventional panoramic view, or at × 60 if placed in contact. The offset turret lens provides magnifications of × 20 and × 150. Light is directed from one lens to the other by means of a proximal button. It is equipped with a focusing wheel.

External sheaths and ancillary instruments

External sheaths may be used for simple diagnostic purposes, carry channels for the passage of ancillary instruments, or have the instruments incorporated as integral parts of the sheath.

Diagnostic sheaths

The microcolpohysteroscope and other small diameter hysteroscopes can be fitted into a diagnostic sheath of small diameter. These sheaths are made of stainless steel, have a medium-tight locking mechanism into which the telescope fits, and are equipped with a single inflow stopcock.

Operative sheaths for the passage of ancillary instruments, and the ancillary instruments

Both the microcolpohysteroscope and the conventional telescopes can be fitted into operative sheaths. Most are equipped with two inflow/outflow stopcocks. A second channel is provided to permit passage of the ancillary instruments. Access to this channel is through a valve which is provided with a rubber nipple for maintaining media-tight integrity. Some sheaths possess a distally situated deflector which is controlled by a proximally sited wheel. It can be used to manipulate the tip of the ancillary instrument into less accessible areas of the uterine cavity. Ancillary instruments may be:
• flexible;
• semi-rigid;
• rigid.
A wide range of biopsy forceps, grasping forceps, scissors, electrodes and probes are available. Most surgeons prefer to use the heavier rigid instruments. Laser fibres can be used with these sheaths.

Sheaths which incorporate the instruments

Two types are used:
• the integral operating sheath;
• the modified urological resectoscope.
Integral sheaths are constructed in such a way that distally placed scissor blades which protrude from the tip of the sheath are controlled by proximally placed handles. The telescope fits into the sheath. The telescope and integral sheath are passed through an external sheath which is equipped with medium inflow and outflow stopcocks. As these instruments are of greater diameter than the diagnostic hysteroscope, the external sheath comes equipped with an obturator. The external sheath and obturator are used to traverse the cervical canal, the obturator is withdrawn and the integral sheath and telescope are inserted.

The modified urological resectoscope is by far the most versatile piece of equipment for the performance of operative hysteroscopy (Fig. 2.4). It is constructed as follows:
• The telescope forms the innermost element.
• The working element (Fig. 2.5), controlled by a proximal grip. This may be equipped with a cylinder or ball electrode, cutting loop, or knife (Figs 2.6 & 2.7).
• The internal sheath, which possesses a ceramic tip and through which is passed the distension medium.

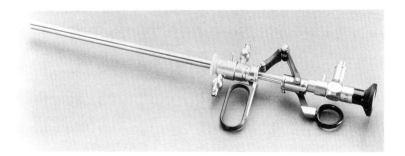

Fig. 2.4 Passive resectoscope.

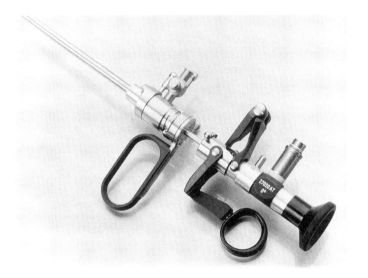

Fig. 2.5 The working element.

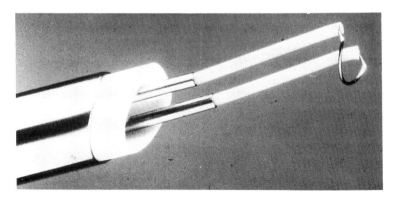

Fig. 2.6 The distal tip of the resectoscope with a 7 mm loop.

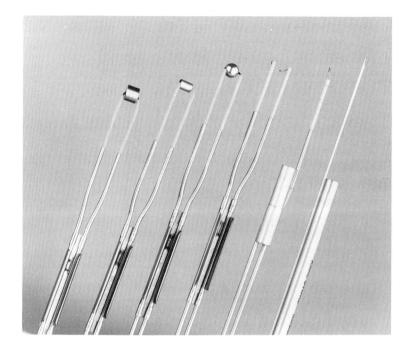

Fig. 2.7 Resectoscope electrodes, left to right: roller cylinder (two), roller ball, resectoscope loop, electric knife (two).

• The stainless steel external sheath, through which the distension medium is evacuated.
• An obturator is provided.

There are two types of working mechanisms, the active and the passive. The element of the active protrudes from the sheath at rest and requires that the surgeon draw it in by pulling the trigger. Conversely, in the passive the surgeon must advance the element by pulling the trigger. Return to the sheath is automatic when the pressure on the trigger is relaxed.

Accidental burns are more easily caused with the former if the electrode is inadvertently activated.

Illumination system

Illumination is provided from an external light source and is transmitted through fibre-optic or fluid-filled cables which are attached to a light post on the proximal end of the hysteroscope. Light sources are available which range from the simple to the complex. The simplest, which is entirely satisfactory for all routine hysteroscopy, has a power of 150 watts. More procedures are being performed by

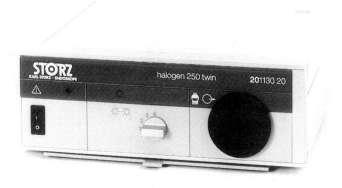

Fig. 2.8 250 watt halogen light source.

observing camera-transmitted images on a television monitor. A
xenon or halogen light source of at least 250 watts is essential if a
video camera is to be used (Fig. 2.8). For those wishing to produce
still photographs an external flash generator is available.

Energy system

Operating procedures will be carried out using:
1 electrosurgical generators; and
2 lasers
as the source of energy.

Electrosurgical generators

Solid state electrosurgical generators (Fig. 2.9) are used which can
deliver, at various wattage outputs, currents in the:
- cutting;
- coagulating; and
- blended modes.

Cutting is effected by rapidly heating the cells so that the intracellular
water explodes. A continuous sine wave current is used. Coagulation
occurs when pulsed current literally cooks the tissue. The currents
can be mixed (blended) to achieve varying degrees of cutting and
coagulation simultaneously. All generators must be compatible with

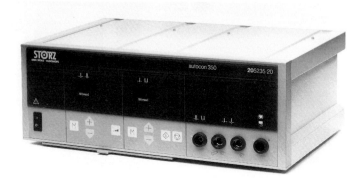

Fig. 2.9 Electrosurgical generator.

the surgical equipment and be equipped with cables to transmit the energy.

Lasers

Laser light is coherent, collimated and monochromatic. 'Coherent' implies that the light waves are exactly synchronized in space and time. 'Collimated' expresses the concept that the light waves are virtually parallel to each other. 'Monochromatic' refers to the uniform colour which occurs because the light waves are all of the same wavelength and hence possess identical quanta of energy. These beams are focused. The neodymium : yttrium aluminium garnet (Nd : YAG) laser has a wavelength of 1.064 µm, and is ideal for hysteroscopic use because it destroys tissue to a depth of 4–6 mm only.

The energy is generated by an external unit and transmitted through a fibre-optic cable with which, if the tip of the cable is left bare, coagulation can be performed. A sapphire tip fitted to the cable tip transforms it into a cutting instrument. The carbon dioxide laser is not suitable for hysteroscopic use because its energy is absorbed by the fluid medium. Furthermore, no satisfactory flexible delivery system is yet available. Neither the potassium titanyl phosphate (KTP) nor the argon lasers possess a deep enough power of penetration.

Documentation

The findings of any hysteroscopic procedure must be recorded. This may be achieved by:
1 a written description;
2 a line drawing;

3 still photography; and

4 videography.

Written description

Immediately after conclusion of each procedure the findings should be recorded in writing. These handwritten or dictated notes will

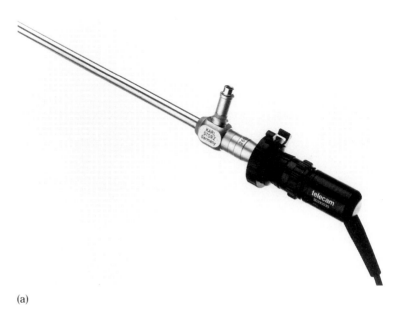

(a)

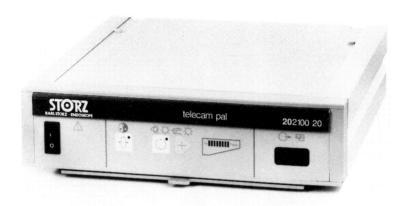

(b)

Fig. 2.10 (a) Silicone chip camera, (b) camera control unit.

form part of the permanent record. For medico–legal purposes they should be as detailed as possible. They should describe the technique, findings and any untoward results. Any recommendations for further management are noted.

Line drawings

It is very helpful to include in the chart a line drawing which may be hand-drawn or filled in on a pre-printed form.

Still photography

Reflex cameras with a focal length varying from $f70$ to $f140$ can be attached to the telescope with a special ring. If it is necessary to take microphotographs through the microcolpohysteroscope a focal length doubler will be required. A cable attaches the shutter release mechanism to the flash generator.

Table 2.1 Equipment required for hysteroscopy

Equipment	Essential	Optional
Distension media and methods of delivery	Carbon dioxide insufflator Glycine Automated pump	Saline Dextrose Hyskon Sorbitol
Telescopes	A conventional telescope compatible with: operative sheaths, integral sheaths, the resectoscope	Microcolpohysteroscope (for *in situ* cytology)
Sheaths	The resectoscope Sheath for ancillary instruments	Integral sheaths
Ancillary instruments	Scissors, biopsy forceps, grasping forceps, electrode	Laser fibre
Illumination system	Cold light source, cables	Xenon light source
Energy system	Solid state generator, cables	Nd : YAG laser
Documentation	Written record, line drawing, video equipment	Still camera

Videography

Remarkable advances in silicone chip technology have resulted in the development of silicone chip cameras which can weigh as little as 130 g (Fig. 2.10, p. 13). Most are equipped with a zoom lens and focusing features. Many cameras must be 'taught' to recognize white by aiming at a white gauze swab. The picture can be displayed on a television monitor, from which many surgeons now operate, and/or stored on the magnetic tape contained in the video recorder. Video cameras are available which direct all the light to the video system. Others are equipped with a beam splitter so that direct observation of the uterine cavity can be made with the naked eye simultaneously with the picture appearing on the screen. Although these cameras are expensive, they are no less integral to the performance of hysteroscopic surgery than the hysteroscope itself. They provide magnification, allow the surgeon to operate in comfort, and are indispensable for the training of others.

Conclusions

It is not the purpose of this chapter to recommend one particular manufacturer's equipment. The list in Table 2.1 (p. 14) should serve to indicate the basic set-up with which all hysteroscopy can be performed appropriately and safely. Equipment may be regarded as essential or optional.

3: Diagnostic Hysteroscopy

Introduction

Diagnostic panoramic hysteroscopy is indicated when direct observation of the uterine cavity is the next step which will either finalize the diagnosis or define the subsequent course of management. Microcolpohysteroscopy can be used to perform colposcopic and microscopic evaluations of the squamo-columnar junction of the cervix.

The technique of diagnostic panoramic hysteroscopy

Any discussion of the technique of diagnostic hysteroscopy must consider:
1 timing;
2 the setting;
3 assembling the equipment;
4 positioning the patient;
5 anaesthesia;
6 introduction of the instruments; and
7 the diagnostic survey.

Timing

Diagnostic panoramic hysteroscopy is an invasive procedure. As a general rule (depending upon the indication for which it is being performed) it should be carried out once the simpler non-invasive tests have been completed. With respect to timing within the menstrual cycle, examinations performed in the follicular phase will yield better information. The endometrium is less lush and there is no risk of inadvertently disturbing a luteal phase pregnancy. It is also better to avoid the immediately pre-ovulatory phase. The copious mucus can be a potent source of intra-uterine bubbles which will hinder observation.

The setting

The setting in which diagnostic hysteroscopy is performed will depend upon the availability of equipment in an out-patient clinic, whether no, local, or general anaesthesia is to be used, whether laparoscopy is to be performed concurrently, and whether it is anticipated that minor or major hysteroscopic procedures are to be undertaken at the same time. Usually the availability of equipment in out-patients, no or local anaesthetic use, and the likelihood that only minor operative procedures will be performed would predicate an out-patient setting. The operating room is the appropriate place if equipment is only available there or if the use of general anaesthesia, the performance of concurrent laparoscopy, or major operative procedures are anticipated.

Assembling the equipment

If diagnostic procedures are to be performed in the unanaesthetized patient it is a simple courtesy to have all in readiness before placing her in the utterly undignified lithotomy position. This preparedness will also reduce the time spent under general anaesthesia for those who require it. All drapes, gowns, and sterile solutions should be ready. The basic diagnostic set-up will include a speculum, swab holder, single-toothed tenaculum, the hysteroscope and sheath, illumination system, distension medium and, where available, video equipment.

A set of cervical dilators should be available but are rarely required for use during diagnostic hysteroscopy. The syringe and needle should be assembled and any local anaesthetic solution to be used drawn up into the syringe.

The hysteroscope should be inserted into the sheath and the lock ring closed. The distension system is connected to the inflow stop-cock and the sheath flushed through to demonstrate easy passage of the medium and that the delivery system is working properly. The tip of the hysteroscope and sheath should be immersed in sterile saline if carbon dioxide is being used. A stream of bubbles will confirm that there is no obstruction to the flow of the gas. If no bubbles appear, the instruments should be disassembled and flushed through with saline. The light cable is attached to the light post of the telescope and the cold light switched on. The telescope is examined to ensure that the lens system is intact and working. If a video camera is to be used it is draped, connected to the lens and focused on a white surface so that the camera can be 'taught' to recognize the colour white. The zoom and focus equipment is tested.

Positioning the patient

Hysteroscopy is carried out with the patient in the dorsal lithotomy position. If awake she is asked to place her feet in the stirrups. Sterile draping is not required but the surgeon should wash and wear gloves. If a television monitor is to be used it should be positioned in such a way that the patient is able to observe the procedure. An assistant who will keep the patient company exerts a calming influence.

If the patient is to be anaesthetized, induction is completed. The patient's lower limbs are placed in the lithotomy stirrups, care being taken to avoid pressure on any of the nerves of the leg. Her hands must be clear of any moving parts of the operating table.

Anaesthesia

The great majority of cases of diagnostic hysteroscopy performed with the smaller bore hysteroscopes using carbon dioxide will not require any anaesthetic. Administration of a prostaglandin syn-thetase inhibitor one hour pre-operatively will reduce any uterine cramping to an absolute minimum. If the patient does experience discomfort, or if a hysteroscope, the insertion of which requires prior cervical dilatation, is required, paracervical blockade can be effected. The local anaesthetic agent of choice is Xylocaine (1%) mixed with 1 IU of ornithine 8 vasopressin (POR 8) in 6–10 ml of saline, with a maximum dosage of 5 IU. Initially 1.5 ml is injected into the cervix at twelve o'clock. To ensure that there is no allergic or hypersensitivity response the surgeon waits for a few moments. Two millilitres are injected into each uterosacral ligament and a further 1 ml into the cervix at three, six and nine o'clock. The depth of injection is 2 cm. As will be described later, certain minor operative procedures can be performed under such local anaesthesia.

If a general anaesthetic is required for technical reasons, or in the very apprehensive patient, the nature of the agents to be used falls within the purview of the anaesthetist.

Introduction of the instruments

Introduction of the small bore diagnostic hysteroscope, which uses carbon dioxide, and the standard diagnostic telescopes, used in conjunction with fluid media, share some aspects of technique. In others they differ. The shared and particular aspects will be described.

Shared aspects of technique

The bladder must be empty. A bimanual examination is performed to evaluate the size and position of the uterus. This will protect the patient against the inadvertent perforation of a retroverted uterus. It also serves to confirm that the bladder is empty. The cervix is exposed. There is no need to introduce antiseptic solutions into the vagina. Passage of the swab causes unnecessary discomfort, and the solution may foul the lens and be a source of bubbles. It is advantageous to cleanse the external os with a small pledget of gauze which is soaked in saline and held in a pair of long forceps. In the unanaesthetized patient a duck-billed speculum, and in the anaesthetized a weighted Auvard type is used. In the latter case, in order to prevent the weighted speculum from slipping from the vagina, a small amount of Trendelenburg position is advisable. Forceful application of the weight to the toes of the surgeon, while being a source of amusement in the otherwise dull day of the nursing staff, may well ensure that the surgeon never dances again.

A single-toothed tenaculum is applied to the cervix in the vertical position. If the patient who is awake is asked to cough just as the tenaculum is applied it is gratifying to note how painlessly the manoeuvre is achieved. From this point the particulars of the techniques diverge.

Small bore hysteroscopes

The use of carbon dioxide with a small bore hysteroscope is the key to the atraumatic, bloodless and pain free dilatation of the cervical canal. The right-handed operator holds the tenaculum in the left hand. With the gas flowing, the tip of the hysteroscope is placed in the external os. The speculum is removed. The pressure of the gas creates a small cavity just in front of the tip of the hysteroscope.

Using either direct vision or the video screen this cavity is identified. It must be remembered that the distal lens is set at an angle of 30°. If the cavity is seen in the middle of the field of vision, the tip of the telescope will be impinging upon the anterior wall of the cervical canal (Fig. 3.1a). The gas-filled cavity must be kept at the bottom of the field of observation (Fig. 3.1b). The telescope is advanced gently as the gas creates a passage at successively higher levels of the cervical canal (Fig. 3.1c). This advance must be unhurried and performed delicately.

If resistance is encountered, or if the surgeon loses sight of the canal, the telescope should be withdrawn for a few millimetres until the cavity reforms. Trying to force the telescope through will produce pain, bleeding which will obscure the field, and may even result in uterine perforation. Once the internal os is passed a few moments waiting will allow the uterine cavity to be distended. If bubbles have formed due to the presence of blood or cervical mucus within the uterine cavity this waiting period generally allows them to dissipate.

Occasionally a very flaccid uterus will allow gas to escape. In these circumstances the flow rate should be reduced to 10 ml/minute. If the cervix is very patulous it may be necessary to place a second tenaculum in such a way as to close the external os around the hysteroscope.

Standard diagnostic hysteroscope

Cervical dilatation is required before insertion of the hysteroscope. As this will inevitably produce bleeding, carbon dioxide is an unsuitable distension medium. Bubbles due to the blood often obscure the field of view. Hyskon is ideal for the very reason that it does not mix with blood. Care must be taken to ensure that any ancillary stopcock is shut. An eyeful of Hyskon will glue the eyelids together. The surgeon's discomfort will once again alleviate the boredom of the nursing staff but serves little other useful purpose.

The cervix is dilated to a size of dilator just smaller than that of the hysteroscope. The system is flushed through with the fluid to remove any air bubbles, and the hysteroscope inserted into the external os. The speculum is removed. The instrument is advanced to the level of the internal os under direct vision. If a clear passage cannot be identified, no attempt should be made to force the instrument forwards. If the lens is obscured, particularly by a red colour, this may be blood or may indicate that the tip of the instrument is impinging on the uterine wall. Perforation of the uterus can too easily occur. The hysteroscope should be withdrawn and cleaned.

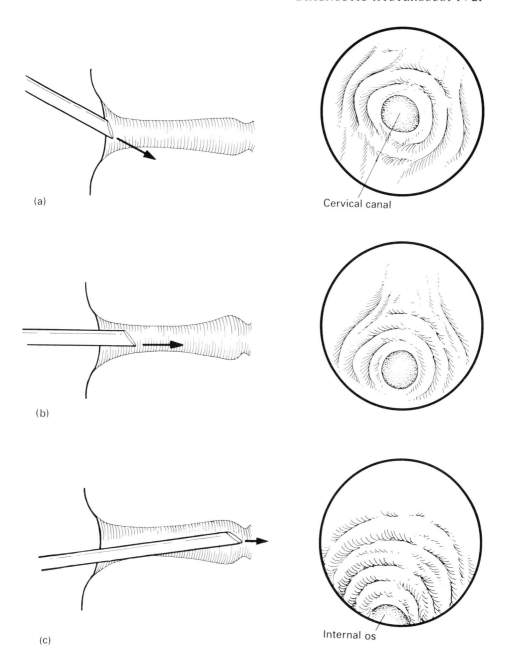

Cervical canal

Internal os

(a)

(b)

(c)

Fig. 3.1 (a) The appearance of the cervical canal in the centre of the field of vision indicates that the tip of the 30° telescope is pointing towards the posterior wall of the canal. (b) The telescope is correctly aligned: the canal is at six o'clock. (c) If the tip of the telescope is used to dilate the internal os, the canal appears below six o'clock.

Occasionally blood in the cavity will obscure the view. If the tip of the telescope is advanced carefully to the fundus or into one cornu the bloody Hyskon will escape and be replaced with clear fluid.

The diagnostic survey

Irrespective of the instrument used, once the uterine cavity has been entered a systematic survey should be performed. The right tubal ostium provides the first landmark (Fig. 3.2). Flow of blood or Hyskon into the tube can be used as a guide to its position if a fluid medium is used. Once the ostium has been identified the hystero-scope is placed in close proximity and the proximal few millimetres of the tube are evaluated (Fig. 3.3) The instrument is withdrawn for a few centimetres and the fundus is observed from right to left until the left ostium is identified. It is scrutinized in a similar fashion to the

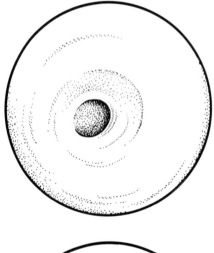

Fig. 3.2 The right tubal ostium seen from mid-cavity.

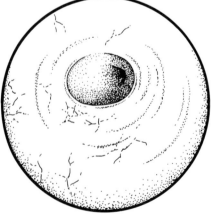

Fig. 3.3 The right tubal ostium showing the proximal portion of the intramural segment.

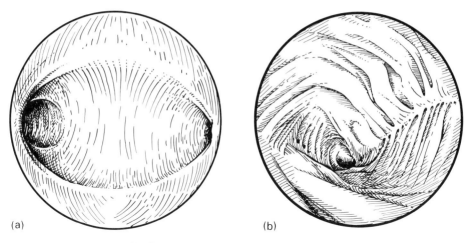

(a)   (b)

Fig. 3.4 (a) The uterine cavity in panoramic view from the internal cervical os; (b) the cervical canal at × 20 magnification.

right. The anterior, lateral and finally posterior walls are evaluated by withdrawing, rotating and advancing the hysteroscope. If the telescope is rotated the 30° distal lens allows otherwise inaccessible areas of the uterus to be seen clearly. Finally withdrawing it to the level of the internal os allows a complete panoramic observation of the entire uterine cavity to be performed (Fig. 3.4a). The cervical canal is evaluated as the telescope is slowly withdrawn (Fig. 3.4b).

If the indication for the diagnostic evaluation was abnormal uterine bleeding and it is proposed to perform hysteroscopic endometrial ablation at a later date, the uterus should be sounded once the hysteroscopy has been completed. Evaluating the length of the cavity by hysteroscopic means alone is extremely difficult. The depth of the uterine cavity has implications for the likelihood of success of endometrial ablation.

Immediately the survey has been completed the findings should be recorded both in writing and on a pictorial hand-drawn or pre-printed sketch of the uterus (Fig. 3.5).

Indications for diagnostic hysteroscopy

Diagnostic panoramic hysteroscopy is indicated in many cases of:
1 abnormal uterine bleeding;
2 infertility and habitual abortion;
3 misplaced intra-uterine contraceptive devices;
4 endometrial carcinoma;
5 previous uterine scars; and
6 following uterine surgery.

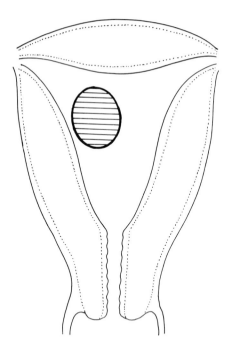

Fig. 3.5 Schematic representation of the uterine cavity with a small fibroid.

Abnormal uterine bleeding

This is the commonest indication for diagnostic hysteroscopy. It should replace diagnostic curettage which may fail to identify up to 25% of causative lesions. If other pelvic pathology is suspected, laparoscopy should be performed concurrently with the hysteroscopy.

Infertility and habitual abortion

The hysterosalpingogram (HSG) remains the preliminary screening test of the tubal and uterine architecture in cases of infertility. If it is abnormal with respect to the uterine cavity, the exact nature of the abnormality should be ascertained hysteroscopically. This will allow a firm diagnosis to be made, a minor procedure performed or any necessary surgery planned. If the HSG reveals a normal uterine cavity, calculations based upon the sensitivity and specificity of the HSG and the known prevalence of uterine lesions in infertile patients would suggest that routine hysteroscopy would be required in 100 such patients in order to identify one abnormality.

If it is unclear whether or not occlusion at the level of the tubo-cornual junction exists, selective hysteroscopic tubal catheterization and chromopertubation at the time of laparoscopy may be of value. A falloposcope can also be introduced at this time.

Uterine lesions may contribute to habitual abortion. When in the course of the investigation of such couples it is deemed appropriate to seek such lesions, diagnostic hysteroscopy should replace hystero-salpingography. It provides an instant diagnosis upon which further treatment can be based. In those patients in whom a congenital malformation is identified, hysteroscopy cannot differentiate be-tween a septate and a bicornuate uterus. Under these circumstances the external configuration of the uterus must be determined laparo-scopically. In the future, imaging techniques may become superior to both laparoscopy and hysteroscopy for the identification of uterine anomalies.

Misplaced intra-uterine contraceptive devices

To determine whether or not an intra-uterine contraceptive device (IUCD) or other foreign body remains within the uterus, simple out-patient hysteroscopy is the initial investigation of choice. Either the IUCD will be identified wholly within the uterine cavity, partly within the cavity and partly embedded in the uterine wall, or the uterus will be noted to be empty. In the last situation a straight X-ray which covers the entire abdomen should be taken. Translocated devices can be found as far away as under the diaphragm. Devices lying wholly within the cavity can be removed immediately. Those embedded within the uterine wall may require more extensive surgery.

Endometrial carcinoma

Pre-cancerous endometrial hyperplasia and areas of frank neoplasia can be identified by visually directed biopsies. Such a step is imperative prior to any contemplated endometrial ablation. It re-mains to be seen whether or not hysteroscopic visualization and directed biopsies in cases of frank invasive uterine cancer will replace fractional curettage.

Previous uterine scars

Investigation of a uterine scar following myomectomy or Caesarean section is sometimes necessary before the patient embarks upon a pregnancy. The degree of fibrosis and depth of any defect can be readily assessed.

Following uterine surgery

Edometrial ablation or resection, excision of a septum, or myomectomy performed hysteroscopically may induce intra-uterine adhesion formation. Formal surgical myomectomy which has involved the uterine cavity and major uterine re-unification procedures may have the same effect. A second look hysteroscopy can be performed six weeks post-operatively to identify and deal with such adhesions.

Contra-indications to hysteroscopy

Although diagnostic hysteroscopy is a safe procedure in expert hands, there are well defined contra-indications which include:
1 infection;
2 cardiorespiratory disease;
3 metabolic acidosis;
4 pregnancy;
5 uterine bleeding;
6 cervical malignancy;
7 cervical stenosis; and
8 the inexperienced surgeon.

Infection

Vaginitis and cervicitis are absolute contra-indications to hysteroscopy because of the danger of causing an ascending infection which may lead to salpingitis or peritonitis. Investigative procedures should be delayed until the infection has been eradicated. For the same reason, hysteroscopy should be avoided in suspected pelvic inflammatory disease. The only exception is infection in the presence of a 'lost' IUCD where hysteroscopy may be necessary to locate and remove it. This procedure should be performed under antibiotic cover.

Cardiorespiratory disease

In severe cardiorespiratory diseases, the use of carbon dioxide as the distension medium may cause gas embolism. The risk has probably been under-reported because of the high solubility of carbon dioxide and the consequent difficulty in substantiating the diagnosis.

Metabolic acidosis

Metabolic acidosis should always be corrected before any surgical procedure, including hysteroscopy, is performed.

Pregnancy

Pregnancy is generally considered a contra-indication to hysteroscopy but it may be necessary to perform hysteroscopy to remove an IUCD (Fig. 3.6), or to diagnose retained products of conception where there has been persistent post-abortal bleeding, although ultrasound has replaced endoscopy in many such cases. The myometrium in the gravid uterus is much more distensible than in the non-pregnant organ which has a strong, resistant muscular wall. Uterine distension with gas can cause the uterus to distend like a balloon resulting in a depot of carbon dioxide accumulating which may lead to separation of the placenta and retroplacental bleeding. The accumulated gas may then flow as a bolus into the ruptured uterine veins causing a massive gas embolus. It is important, therefore, that hysteroscopy in pregnancy is only performed by an expert surgeon who is aware of these possibilities and that the gas flow is restricted to 20 ml/minute with an intra-uterine pressure of less than 50 mmHg. It is also important to remember that the optic nerve of the fetus may be damaged by the hysteroscope light after the tenth week of pregnancy, although there does not appear to be any danger before this stage.

Uterine bleeding

Scanty or moderate uterine bleeding does not prevent adequate observation of the uterine cavity but heavy bleeding will prevent clear visualization regardless of the distension medium used. Heavy bleeding should usually be suppressed to allow full evaluation of the endometrium and prevent intravasation of the distension medium.

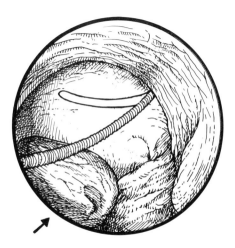

Fig. 3.6 IUCD in a uterus with an early pregnancy sac.

Despite this there have been reports of hysteroscopy being performed during persistent heavy bleeding episodes and haemorrhagic areas of the endometrium coagulated to control it. If it is imperative that hysteroscopy be performed during such a bleeding episode the only effective instrument is a double channel continuous flow hysteroscope. The pressure of the distension fluid will often be sufficient to arrest the bleeding and allow the residual blood to be flushed.

Hysteroscopy should be avoided during menstruation, not only because of a theoretical risk of dissemination of endometriosis but mainly because the view is usually unsatisfactory.

Cervical carcinoma

Hysteroscopy should not be performed in the presence of occult or overt cervical carcinoma because of the danger of disseminating malignant cells. The situation here differs from that of endometrial carcinoma. There is no evidence that there is any spread of malignant endometrial cells. In cases of invasive carcinoma of the cervix there is a very real risk that passage of the telescope may open blood or lymphatic vessels and cause systemic dissemination.

Cervical stenosis

The risk of uterine perforation is considerably greater in such patients. It may be necessary to proceed with extreme caution or on occasions simply decide not to attempt to perform the procedure.

The inexperienced surgeon

'Watch one, do one, teach one' is no longer an acceptable standard of practice. Those wishing to perform diagnostic hysteroscopy must undergo a period of formal training (see Chapter 8).

Complications of diagnostic hysteroscopy

Diagnostic hysteroscopy is a safe procedure when performed correctly for the proper indications by a well-trained surgeon. As with any invasive technique, there may be complications. In 1986, H.-J. Lindemann carried out a postal survey of the experience of European hysteroscopists and found the incidence of serious complications to be 0.012%. In addition there were a number of minor complications, but no deaths were recorded. It must be remembered that all the surgeons involved in this survey were expert hysteroscopists. The complications of diagnostic hysteroscopy are:

1 failure to complete the procedure;
2 those due to the distension medium;
3 those due to the procedure; and
4 those due to anaesthesia.

Failure to complete the procedure

This event should occur in less than 2% of patients and can be accounted for by failure to dilate the cervix, bubbles of blood or mucus in the cavity, the occasional case of severe discomfort in the non-anaesthetized patient, and inexperience of the surgeon.

The distension medium

Carbon dioxide may cause post-operative shoulder tip pain. A death has been reported following the use of an inappropriate type of insufflator. If the proper equipment is used gas embolism with carbon dioxide is unlikely to occur during diagnostic hysteroscopy because the procedure should be fairly brief and the volume of gas used should not exceed 200–400 ml. Embolism is probably under-diagnosed because carbon dioxide is so soluble in tissue fluids and is absorbed before the occurrence of embolism can be proven.

High molecular weight dextran

A very few cases of anaphylaxis or adult onset respiratory distress syndrome have been reported.

Other fluid media

Carbon dioxide, high molecular weight dextran, and the other fluid media may all cause rupture of thin-walled hydrosalpinges. Fluid overload, which is a major problem in operative hysteroscopy, should be rare during diagnostic procedures because: the duration should be short, the volume of fluid used should be small, and the uterine vessels should not be ruptured to allow intravasation of fluid.

The procedure

Cervical trauma, uterine perforation, and activation of acute pelvic inflammatory disease may occur.

Cervical trauma

The most frequent complication of diagnostic hysteroscopy is trauma caused by the instruments. It is unusual to need to dilate the cervix except in the post-menopausal woman or, less commonly, in the nulliparous patient. It is preferable to use the passive dilatation produced by the carbon dioxide to permit atraumatic introduction of the hysteroscope. If the cervix has to be dilated then there may be laceration by the cervical tenaculum, and the dilators frequently produce bleeding from vessels in the cervical canal. Bleeding from a tenaculum puncture site or laceration may be controlled by pressure applied with ring forceps or may require sutures.

Uterine perforation

Uterine perforation is unlikely to occur if the hysteroscope is passed under continuous direct vision. Perforation during diagnostic hysteroscopy does not usually produce side-effects and can be treated conservatively.

Pelvic inflammatory disease

A very small number of patients may show evidence of acute pelvic inflammatory disease 24–48 hours after diagnostic hysteroscopy. The occurrence of this event can be kept to an absolute minimum by remembering the contra-indications. If it should occur, management is by intensive antibiotic administration, based upon the results of bacteriological studies.

Anaesthesia

Idiosyncratic or allergic reactions can occur with the use of local anaesthetic agents. Those complications of general anaesthesia, which fortunately are exceedingly rare, do not differ from those when a general anaesthetic is administered for any minor surgical procedure.

The normal and abnormal hysteroscopic appearances

The normal uterine cavity, when distended, is ovoid in the coronal plane. The contour is regular and smooth. The fundus is slightly convex and is often misinterpreted as being arcuate. The cornua are seen as darker recesses at two and ten o'clock. This is the picture usually seen as the internal os is passed (see Fig. 3.4a). When the telescope is advanced into the cornu the tubal ostia will be noted. There is much variance in the depth of the cornua. There may be a partial annular membrane behind which the tubal ostium will be seen (Fig. 3.7a). The ostium may initially be closed and appear as a slit (Fig. 3.7b). As the pressure of the gas increases, the ostium will open and assume a circular configuration. It may be seen to open and close in a rhythmic fashion. Normal follicular phase endo-metrium is pink or tan in colour. Few blood vessels will be observed. A similar appearance will be noted in the post-menopausal woman. Secretory phase endometrium is thicker, velvety and pink or tan. Small blood vessels can be observed with ease. The thickness of the tissue can be estimated by creating a furrow in the posterior surface with the tip of the hysteroscope (Fig. 3.8). The panoramic hystero-scope permits accurate identification of:

1 polyps;
2 fibroids;
3 adhesions;
4 septa;
5 adenomyosis;
6 uterine scars;
7 heterotopic bone;
8 endometrial hyperplasia; and
9 adenocarcinoma.

Each will be described and its relevance to the presenting symptom which constituted the indication for the diagnostic hysteroscopy will be discussed.

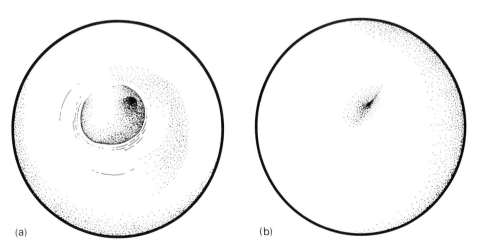

(a) (b)

Fig. 3.7 (a) The partial annular membrane with the tubal ostium open; (b) closed tubal ostium without a significant membrane.

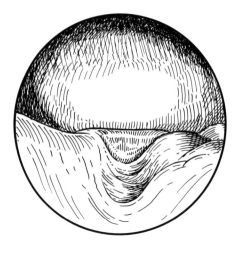

Fig. 3.8 Groove formed by the tip of the hysteroscope indicating the thickness of the endometrium.

Polyps

Polyps may be mucous or fibrous. Mucous polyps may be single or multiple, sessile or pedunculated (Fig. 3.9). Their colour is similar to that of the surrounding endometrium. Fibrous polyps are usually pedunculated, smooth, firm and poorly vascularized. Such polyps may be of significance in cases of abnormal bleeding. They are otherwise incidental findings.

Fibroids

Large intra-mural fibroids may distort the regular contour of an otherwise normal uterine cavity. Submucous lesions are either sessile or pedunculated (Fig. 3.10). The covering endometrium is

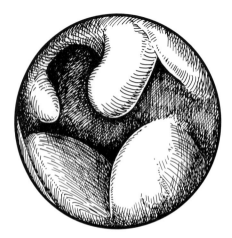

Fig. 3.9 Multiple mucous polyps.

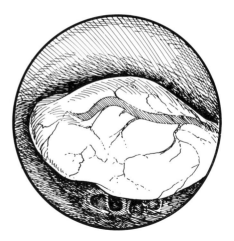

Fig. 3.10 Pedunculated submucous myoma.

pale coloured. There may be obvious surface blood vessels. They are a potent source of abnormal bleeding, and may be associated with habitual abortion but do not cause infertility.

Adhesions

These are classified in order of severity as endometrial, fibro-muscular and fibrous. They may be situated laterally or centrally within the cavity (Fig. 3.11). They have a typical pale appearance. The more severe the degree of adhesion formation, the greater the diminution of menstrual flow. Those found in eumenorrhoeic infertile patients are incidental findings. Those causing hypo- or amenorrhoea may cause infertility or be associated with habitual abortion.

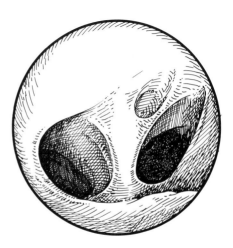

Fig. 3.11 Intra-uterine adhesions.

Septa

Septa may be complete, that is extending to the cervical canal, or incomplete. As the hysteroscope traverses the cervix the dark areas of the two hemi-uteri will be seen divided by a pale partition (Fig. 3.12). Each hemi-cavity possesses only one tubal ostium. The medially placed septum is usually paler than the surrounding normal endometrium. Septa do not cause infertility but may be associated with habitual abortion.

Adenomyosis

Occasionally hypervascularization associated with raised, dark, sub-mucous blebs may be noted. Adenomyosis should be suspected. It is a cause of abnormal bleeding.

Uterine scars

The dimensions and characteristics of any uterine scars are usually obvious.

Heterotopic bone

Rare cases may be noted. They usually occur following abortion. The bony fragments are white or yellow and may be fan- or disc-shaped. Small, specific bones such as the humerus may be identified. The presence of this bone may cause infertility.

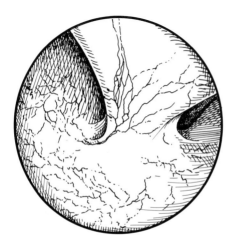

Fig. 3.12 A complete uterine septum extending almost to the cervical canal.

Endometrial hyperplasia

Benign cystic and adenomatous hyperplasia do not have typical panoramic hysteroscopic appearances. The endometrium may appear to be excessively thick if a furrow is created. The diagnosis is made by hysteroscopically directed biopsy. Both lesions may be encountered in cases of abnormal uterine bleeding.

Adenocarcinoma

The lesions may be circumscribed or diffuse. They may affect the corpus or extend to within the cervical canal. They are vegetative and frequently necrotic, friable and hypervascular. They bleed easily if touched. They may be associated with collections of fluid or pus which makes visualization difficult. The presenting symptom will have been peri- or post-menopausal bleeding.

The technique of microcolpohysteroscopy

The microcolpohysteroscope (Hamou 1) is a complex optical telescope which is capable of providing magnifications of $\times 1$, $\times 20$, $\times 60$ and $\times 150$. Carbon dioxide is always used as the distension medium. The ability to make histological examinations *in situ* is valuable in:
1 the cervix; and
2 the uterine cavity.
To perform microcolpohysteroscopy of the cervix or uterine cavity the surgeon will require:
• the telescope and diagnostic sheath;
• a small operative sheath for the passage of ancillary instruments;
• biopsy forceps, dye cannulae and (if necessary) minor operative instruments;
• a gas insufflator and gas line;
• a light source and cables;
• fine forceps for carrying cotton swabs;
• saline to cleanse the cervix;
• supravital stains.
The setting (out-patient), assembly of the equipment, positioning of the patient and anaesthesia (usually none, occasionally local) do not vary from when the instrument is used in a panoramic mode. At this point attention must be paid to examination of:
1 the uterus alone;
2 the uterus and cervix; and

3 the cervix alone.

The uterus alone

The uterus should be examined in the follicular phase. Initial evaluation is performed at × 20. One per cent methylene blue can be injected through a polythene cannula to delineate better the glandular structures. A wait of a few minutes allows the dye to become concentrated at the bases of the glands. Examination is then performed at × 150.

The uterus and cervix

If an evaluation of both the uterus and cervix is to be performed the uterus should be examined first. Soiling of the distal lens with debris and mucus will occur if the cervix is examined first.

The cervix alone

Histological evaluation at × 150 can be performed *in situ*. Mid-cycle is best because the cervix is dilated and the mucus watery. The steps of cervical examination are:
1 cleansing and staining;
2 insertion of the hysteroscope;
3 identification of the squamo-columnar junction; and
4 performance of the survey.

Cleansing and staining. The cervix is exposed with the speculum and the tenaculum applied. The cervix is gently cleansed with normal saline. The saline and the stains are applied using cotton wool swabs held in the fine forceps. Lugol's iodine (2%) is applied to the ectocervix and first few millimetres of the endocervix. Iodo-negative areas can be identified and, if necessary, the instrument used as a colposcope at × 20 magnification. Waterman's blue fountain pen ink is brought to a pH of 5. The solution is applied as was the Lugol's iodine.

Insertion of the hysteroscope. The flow rate of carbon dioxide is set at 12–15 ml/minute. Initial observations are performed at a magnification of × 60, with the tip of the telescope in contact with the epithelium. The circumference of the cervical canal is examined by moving the telescope in a circular fashion. Nucleocytoplasmic observation is carried out by pushing the button to divert the image to the offset lens. With the objective still in contact a magnification of × 150 will be obtained. The transformation zone is identified and examined in its entirety.

The endocervix is stained with 1% methylene blue solution. The instrument is advanced to the internal os, magnification set at $\times 60$ and the canal from the os to the squamo-columnar junction is observed.

As can be imagined, small movements of the distal end of the instrument will result in oscillation of the proximal end. To stabilize the telescope a right-handed surgeon should hold the distal end in the right hand and rest the left hand on the perineum, gripping the hysteroscope between the thumb and index finger.

Indications for microcolpohysteroscopy

Microcolpohysteroscopy is indicated for:
1 Evaluation of the cervix as an adjunct to:
  (a) naked eye examination;
  (b) Papanicolaou smears; and
  (c) colposcopy.
Microcolpohysteroscopy has an evolving role in cancer screening.
2 Evaluation of the glandular structure of the endometrium.
In either situation it can be used to identify areas from which directed biopsies should and can be taken.

Contra-indications and complications

1 Overt invasive carcinoma of the cervix;
2 The inexperienced surgeon.
If used within the uterine cavity the complications are those of panoramic hysteroscopy. There are essentially no complications, other than that of making an incorrect diagnosis if the cervix alone is being evaluated.

The indications will not be discussed in detail here but will become apparent when the lesions which can be identified are described.

The normal and abnormal microcolpohysteroscopic findings

This section will describe:
1 the normal uterine findings;
2 the abnormal uterine appearances;
3 the normal cervical findings; and
4 the abnormal cervical findings.

Normal uterine findings

Panoramic appearances have been described. Following staining and examination at × 150 the glandular orifices can be seen as dark blue circles against a light blue background. After a wait of a few moments the tubular nature of the glands can be seen as dark blue culs-de-sac which stand out against the red of the stroma.

Abnormal uterine appearances

Examination at magnification may be of value in case of:
1 polyps;
2 adhesions;
3 endometrial hyperplasia; and
4 endometritis.

Polyps

When examined at × 20 mucous polyps will be identical in appearance to the surrounding endometrium. Fibrous polyps are poorly vascularized. No gland orifices can be noted.

Adhesions

At × 20 endometrial adhesions do not differ from the surrounding tissue. Myofibrous lesions are covered with pale endometrium but the glandular orifices are still identifiable. Such is not the case with fibrous adhesions. They are devoid of any endometrial covering.

Endometrial hyperplasia

Evaluation is performed at × 20 after staining with methylene blue. Glandular openings of up to 1 mm may be seen in cases of cystic hyperplasia. In addition to widened glandular openings, areas of increased vascularization are particularly notable when adenomatous hyperplasia is present. This vascularization becomes particularly disorganized and the glandular openings are squashed together in pre-cancerous hyperplasia.

Endometritis

Staining is not required. At × 20 the endometrium, particularly at the tubal ostia, has an appearance which is similar to cervicitis when viewed colposcopically. The endometrium is bright red and the glandular openings appear as raised white or yellow spots scattered throughout.

Normal cervical findings

From the ectocervix to the cervical canal three areas can be identified:
1 the squamous epithelium (ectocervix);
2 the squamo-columnar junction or transformation zone; and
3 the columnar epithelium (endocervix).

The squamous epithelium

Five layers of cells can be identified:
  (a) basal, small cuboidal cells;
  (b) parabasal, larger polyhedral cells;
  (c) intermediate, there is gradual maturation of the cells with reduction of the size of the nucleus;
  (d) superficial, large polyhedral cells with small nuclei; and
  (e) desquamated, these are loosely-lying superficial cells.
When examined at $\times 20$ or $\times 150$ only the upper two layers can be seen with the microcolpohysteroscope. Normally the glycogen containing cytoplasm is brownish-yellow (Lugol's iodine) and the nuclei dark blue (Waterman's ink).

The squamo-columnar junction

Usually situated at the level of the external os this is the region where the squamous and columnar cells meet. There is gradual exposure of all the layers of the squamous epithelium with the exception of the parabasal. Even these cells may be observed in hypo-estrogenic women. The deeper layers, intermediate and parabasal do not contain glycogen. They will be pale blue with dark blue nuclei. At the junction the columnar cells of the endocervix overlap the squamous cells.

The columnar epithelium

The cells are long, columnar and possess basal nuclei. The tip is filled with mucus. At $\times 20$ the folds of the epithelium are very obvious. At $\times 60$ the invaginations (there are no true glands), called crypts are seen as pale areas the rims of which will stain with methylene blue.

At ×150 the cells and their darker nuclei will be very obvious.

Thus when the normal cervix is evaluated at ×150 from below upwards the observer will note the brownish-yellow superficial squamous epithelium, and the dark blue edge of the intermediate and parabasal cells of the transformation zone, which has a sinuous, clearly demarcated border with the lighter blue columnar cells. The position of the transitional zone and the cellular characteristics of epithelia vary with the age of the patient and the phase of the menstrual cycle.

Abnormal cervical findings

Microcolpohysteroscopic examination may be of value in cases of:
1 metaplasia;
2 mosaicism;
3 inflammation;
4 condylomata;
5 leucoplakia; and
6 dysplasia and cervical intra-epithelial neoplasia (CIN).

Metaplasia

Metaplasia occurs when the columnar cells are exposed to environmental changes. The nuclear DNA becomes exposed to these influences, may incorporate foreign proteins and hence alter the cellular metabolism and physical characteristics. This is a dynamic process which can be observed at ×150 over a time span. Cells undergoing metaplasia in the early stages will lose their mucus and the nuclei will take up Waterman's blue. The previously obvious capillaries become hidden. Islets of normal columnar epithelium will be noted surrounded by metaplastic cells.

Mosaicism

Incomplete metaplasia produces a picture at ×150 of arched dark columnar cells surrounding darker areas of squamous cells. This appearance is termed 'mosaicism'.

Inflammation

At ×20 the red, stippled with yellow dots of cervicitis, is readily seen. At ×150 patches of cells become elongated and may in places be raised above the surface.

Condylomata

Condylomata acuminata may occur on the cervix, in isolation or in conjunction with other dysplastic changes. At ×150 vascular bundles of connective tissue will be noted, between which lie the koilocytes. These are large cells with excessive cytoplasm. The dark stained nuclei are large and irregular and may be polyhedral. The nuclei are never as large as those seen in cases of carcinoma *in situ*.

Leucoplakia

Leucoplakia occurs when keratin forms on the cervix. At ×20 it is seen as thick, white (iodo-negative) plaques. At ×150 the anucleate squamous cells, which do not take up Waterman's blue, are obvious.

Dysplasia and CIN

Pre-cancerous lesions of the cervix are described by the term dysplasia. The ×150 appearances which characterize dysplasia and its most extreme form CIN involve nucleo-cytoplasmic abnormalities which may include the entire thickness of the squamous epithelium. They seem to arise, and are certainly best observed, at the transformation zone.

   Hamou and co-workers have devised a classification of microcolpohysteroscopically observed cervical changes which will be used here. It is as follows:

Grade 0 Indicates normality
Grade 1 Indicates the presence of a dystrophy (infection, metaplasia condylomata, mosaicism) not associated with dysplasia
Grade 2 Indicates the presence of dysplasia and includes carcinoma *in situ*

(Carcinoma *in situ* is a lesion possessing the cytological and histological characteristics of invasive cancer but confined to the surface epithelium. This diagnosis can only be made conclusively at the time of formal histological evaluation of biopsy specimens.)

   The keys to the microcolpohysteroscopic diagnosis of dysplasia are evaluation of:
   (a) nuclear size;
   (b) nuclear colour;
   (c) nuclear shape;
   (d) the nucleocytoplasmic ratio;

(e) other characteristics such as anisokaryosis; and dyschromasia.

Nuclear size. At $\times 150$ normal nuclei of squamous cells are $6\,\mu m$ in diameter. Dysplastic nuclei exceed $15\,\mu m$.

Nuclear colour. Dysplastic nuclei are much darker than normal nuclei. This characteristic is referred to as hyperchromasia.

Nuclear shape. Normal nuclei are round. Dysplastic nuclei are heterogenous in shape.

Nucleocytoplasmic ratio (NCR). Because of the increased size of the dysplastic nucleus relative to the rest of the cell the NCR will be reduced.

Anisokaryosis. This term describes the finding of nuclei of greatly varying size within one field of view.

Dyschromasia. The term used to describe the variation in colour of adjacent nuclei.

In the hands of a hysteroscopist skilled in the recognition of cytological abnormalities, microcolpohysteroscopy is a most valuable adjunct to clinical cytology and colposcopy. When it is recognized that in a significant number of cases the abnormal squamo-columnar junction will not be visible to the colposcopist it can readily be appreciated how microcolpohysteroscopically directed biopsy could save a number of women from the need to undergo a formal cone biopsy.

It was remarked that an evolving indication for microcolpohysteroscopy was in cancer screening. At present the technique must be used as an adjunct to Papanicolaou smears. Nevertheless a growing body of clinical investigation is beginning to show that microcolpohysteroscopy may be as accurate as the smear as a means of dysplasia and early cancer detection and follow-up.

Conclusions

The techniques, indications, contra-indications and complications of panoramic and microcolpohysteroscopy have been described. The normal and abnormal appearances viewed both panoramically and at high magnification have been discussed. The surgeon should become a fully competent diagnostic hysteroscopist before attempting to perform simple operative procedures.

4: Pre-operative Investigation and Management

Introduction

The pre-operative investigation and management of any patient undergoing hysteroscopic surgery should focus upon:
- the general investigation common to all patients;
- the investigation and management which is specific to the presenting symptom.

The general investigation and management

All patients who will be submitted to hysteroscopic surgery have four things in common:

1 they may undergo a general anaesthetic;

2 they may be put at some risk of fluid overload;

3 they may need to be placed in the lithotomy position for an extended time;

4 they will be put at some, albeit small, risk of developing acute pelvic inflammatory disease.

The general investigation should, by history, physical examination and selected laboratory tests identify any pre-existing conditions which might require correction prior to the surgery, or indeed make the surgery contra-indicated. Every endeavour should be made to obtain any previous medical record.

History

Enquiry should be made about:
- general state of health;
- any present illnesses, particularly of the cardiorespiratory, hepatic, or renal systems;
- current medications;
- any tendency to, or active, diabetes;

- current tobacco, alcohol or street drug use;
- drug allergies, particularly to antibiotics;
- any previous anaesthetics. Idiosyncratic reactions and the rare, but potentially lethal, malignant hyperthermia should be sought;
- previous illnesses;
- previous blood transfusions, and reactions if any;
- the possibility that the patient may be pregnant. Failure to discuss the menstrual history, date of last menstrual period, and, where necessary, performance of a pregnancy test can lead to disaster.

General physical examination

The pulse rate and blood pressure should be noted. The cardiovascular and respiratory systems are examined thoroughly. Identification of a cardiac lesion may indicate the need to prescribe prophylactic antibiotics against the risk of bacterial endocarditis.

Patients who suffer from disorders of the musculo-skeletal system should attempt to adopt the lithotomy position to ensure that access can be gained to the pelvic organs. This can be tested when the routine pelvic examination is performed.

In many institutions a pre-anaesthetic service is provided by the anaesthetists. If the general history or physical examination suggests that the patient might be at undue risk from general anaesthesia or fluid absorption, or suffers from a bleeding tendency, consultation should be sought with this service or appropriate specialist if the service is not available.

General laboratory tests

The level of the haemoglobin should be measured. If it is subnormal, surgery should be delayed until the anaemia has been corrected. Routine urinalysis is of little value. If a diabetic tendency is suspected, a fasting blood sugar level should be assessed. Sugar-containing fluid distension media should be avoided in such patients. Many institutions insist that the patient's Australia antigen status be determined so that any necessary intra-operative precautions can be taken. Routine screening for the human immunodeficiency virus is not recommended, although it can be offered to the patient. It is wiser to assume that all patients are infected and operate accordingly. Fortunately hysteroscopists and their surgical teams are not at great risk from needle stab injuries.

Swabs should be taken from the vagina and cervix and sent for bacteriological examination at the time of the pelvic examination.

Any major pathogens detected by this process should be treated with antibiotics prior to even a diagnostic hysteroscopy. If a recent Papanicolaou smear has not been performed this should be carried out.

The investigation and management which is specific to the presenting symptom

Patients undergoing hysteroscopic surgery will be suffering from abnormal bleeding, infertility or habitual abortion. The investigation and management which should be performed prior to complex hysteroscopic surgery for each will be listed.

Abnormal bleeding

- Menstrual history including date of last menstrual period.
- Estimation of blood loss.
- Evaluation of haemoglobin levels.
- Evaluation of thyroid function where indicated.
- Evaluation of any suspected bleeding diathesis.
- Pelvic ultrasound to identify any obvious uterine lesions.

Management

- Specific therapy of any identified non-uterine cause.

Further investigation

- If no non-uterine cause identified.
- If management of non-uterine cause fails.
- Diagnostic hysteroscopy, endometrial biopsy and uterine sounding.

Further management

- If adenomatous hyperplasia or carcinoma *in situ* is detected, endometrial ablation is contra-indicated.
- If the uterus is greater than 10 cm in depth endometrial ablation is unlikely to succeed.
- If the uterus is smaller than 12 cm and the endometrium is benign with no evidence of intra-uterine polyps or fibroids, a trial of non-surgical use of progestational agents or low dose danazol is indicated.

- Hysteroscopic surgery should be performed if:
  (a) non-surgical therapy fails;
  (b) the patient chooses this approach rather than hysterectomy.

Infertility

Investigations

- Menstrual history (ovulatory or anovulatory).
- Semen analysis (normal or abnormal).
- HSG.

Management

The management of infertility is beyond the scope of this text. If however the HSG demonstrates a 'filling defect' of the uterine cavity, simple diagnostic hysteroscopy is indicated to delineate the nature of the lesion.

Habitual abortion

Investigations

- History.
- Evaluation of thyroid and prolactin status.

Management

The management of habitual abortion is beyond the scope of this text. If these simple screening tests are normal, or if correcting them fails to resolve the problem, diagnostic hysteroscopy and endometrial sampling on day 26 should be performed. Uterine lesions believed causative can, in many instances, be treated with hysteroscopic surgery.

5: Simple Operative Procedures

Introduction

It can be argued that the expression 'simple operative procedure' is an oxymoron. The term is used here to denote those hysteroscopic procedures which can be performed in the out-patient department without recourse to general anaesthesia, and include:

1 biopsy of the cervix;
2 biopsy of the endometrium;
3 removal of small single polyps or fibroids;
4 removal of medium-sized single polyps or fibroids;
5 removal of less dense adhesions;
6 removal of non-embedded IUCDs;
7 tubal cannulation; and
8 tubal sterilization.

The basic equipment

The performance of simple surgical procedures requires little in the way of equipment. As most can be carried out at the time of diagnostic hysteroscopy if a lesion is detected, it is wise to have available the appropriate ancillary instruments. Basic equipment should include:

• the hysteroscope and diagnostic sheath;
• a sheath to permit passage of ancillary instruments;
• grasping forceps;
• scissors;
• an electrode and electrosurgical generator, cables and return plate;
• biopsy forceps;
• soft polyethylene cannula;
• the distension system;
• the lighting system;

- a duck-billed speculum;
- a single-toothed tenaculum;
- a paracervical block kit.

All simple operations can be performed using one of the fine bore telescopes, and as bleeding is rarely encountered, carbon dioxide is an excellent distension medium.

Timing

Simple procedures require no special preparation of the endometrium. They are best carried out in the follicular phase. Most will not be planned but will follow as soon as diagnostic hysteroscopy has revealed the presence of a lesion which is amenable to treatment.

Anaesthesia

For the majority of patients diagnostic hysteroscopy will have been performed without anaesthesia. A useful, humane practice is to explain to the patient the nature of the surgery to be performed. If she experiences pain the surgery can be discontinued temporarily and a paracervical block inserted. If such a local anaesthetic was given to facilitate the diagnostic step it will naturally suffice if minor surgery is to be performed.

General anaesthesia is only required if the patient is extremely apprehensive.

The specific operations

Biopsy of the cervix

Special equipment

- Supravital stains (see Chapter 3).
- Microcolpohysteroscope.
- Operative sheath.
- Punch biopsy forceps.

Technique

As multiple biopsies must usually be taken it is advisable to perform paracervical blockade. The cervix is stained (Chapter 3) and the transformation zone identified. In cases of dysplasia or CIN the area or areas with the greatest concentration of abnormal cells are identified at $\times 150$. In cases of dystrophy any areas which should be sampled are identified.

The hysteroscope is withdrawn sufficiently that a panoramic view of the area to be sampled is obtained. The forceps are passed through the operating channel and the punch biopsy taken. The procedure is repeated as often as deemed necessary.

Follow-up

If there is histological evidence of severe dysplasia or CIN a formal cone biopsy must be performed, and further treatment based upon these findings. Lesser degrees of dysplasia or dystrophy may be followed by regular microcolpohysteroscopic evaluations, by further directed biopsies where appropriate, or by classical cytological and colposcopic means.

Complications

Very occasionally, bleeding may occur, either at the time of biopsy or a few days post-operatively. It can be controlled with a simple suture. Cervicitis is prevented by the use of topical antibiotic cream for several days post-operatively.

Biopsy of the endometrium

Equipment

- Standard equipment.
- If microcolpohysteroscopy is performed, methylene blue stain and fine catheter for dye injection.
- Biopsy forceps.
- Novak or similar biopsy curette.

Technique

The endometrium is examined. Biopsies are taken from any suspicious areas under direct vision by simply introducing the forceps, opening the jaws, advancing the forceps and removing tissue by closing the jaws. It has been noted that on occasion the amount of tissue so obtained is not adequate for the pathologist's purposes. It may be more effective to remove the hysteroscope and insert a Novak or similar endometrial biopsy curette towards the area to be sampled, take the sample and reintroduce the hysteroscope to ensure that the tissue has been taken from the correct site. Bleeding often hinders this second examination.

Follow-up

Follow-up will be dependent upon the results of the histological evaluation. Carcinoma of the endometrium will require definitive treatment. Patients complaining of abnormal bleeding in whom adenomatous hyperplasia or carcinoma *in situ* is discovered should not undergo endometrial ablation.

Complications

There are none, other than those associated with diagnostic hysteroscopy.

Removal of small polyps or fibroids

Equipment

- Standard equipment.
- Grasping forceps.
- 5 French electrode.
- Laser and conducting fibres.
- Sorbitol and delivery system.

Technique

Single pedunculated mucous or fibrous polyps of less than 1 cm diameter can be dealt with at the time of diagnostic hysteroscopy by one of these techniques:

1 Grasping forceps can be inserted alongside the hysteroscope and guided to the polyp under direct vision. The polyp is grasped (Fig. 5.1). The hysteroscope is removed and the polyp twisted until it is avulsed. A re-examination is performed to ensure complete removal.

2 The blunt 5 French electrode is inserted and the tip buried in the pedicle at its base (Fig. 5.2). If the tip is not buried smoke will obscure the view. Power (15 watts) is applied until the pedicle blanches. The pedicle is divided with cutting current. This technique is remarkably painless. The polyp will be expelled spontaneously within a few days.

3 A defocused laser can be used to vaporize the polyp. This high-

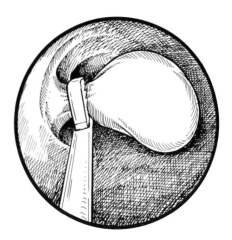

Fig. 5.1 A small pedunculated mucous polyp grasped with semi-rigid forceps.

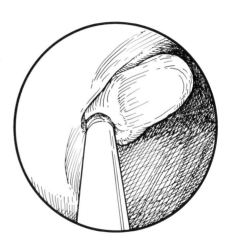

Fig. 5.2 The tip of the electrode is coagulating the base of a pedunculated polyp.

tech approach is somewhat like using a sledgehammer to crack a nut, particularly as the laser can only be used in a fluid medium.

Removal of medium-sized single polyps or fibroids (between 1 and 2 cm)

Equipment

- Dilators and polyp forceps.
- Resectoscope or Nd : YAG laser.
- Fluid distension medium and delivery pump.
- Paracervical block kit.

Technique

The lesion will almost certainly have been identified at the time of diagnostic hysteroscopy. The instrument is removed and a paracervical block inserted. A few moments are allowed to elapse until the block has taken effect. The cervix is dilated and the resectoscope inserted. (For further details see Chapter 3.) The surgeon achieves orientation within the uterine cavity by identifying the tubal ostia. The loop of the resectoscope is passed distally to the lesion (Fig. 5.3). A blended current of 100 watts cutting and 50 watts coagulating is applied and the cutting stroke made. Cutting must *always* be from the direction of the fundus towards the cervix.

Small lesions may be completely removed with only one cutting stroke. If it is necessary to excise the lesion piecemeal, the slices of tissue can simply be pushed into the fundus until the cutting phase has been completed. The resectoscope is taken out and the fragments removed with forceps and sent for histological examination. Any remaining pieces of excised tissue will be expelled spontaneously within a day or two.

If dislodged tissue adheres to the cutting loop, the active element and telescope are disengaged from the external sheath. Withdrawal of these components into the external sheath will remove the lesion. If it becomes necessary to take two or more slices of the lesion by reinserting the resectoscope, it is absolutely vital that the uterus be allowed to redistend prior to applying the electric current.

The Nd : YAG laser can be used to vaporize such polyps or fibroids. The earlier remarks still pertain.

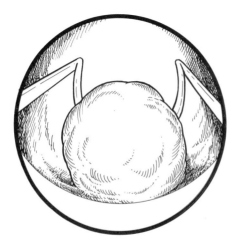

Fig. 5.3 Resection of submucous fibroid.

Follow-up

No adjunctive therapy need be given. An out-patient hysteroscopy is performed 6 weeks post-operatively. Adhesion formation is rare, but should it have occurred the adhesion can be dealt with easily as will be described below.

Complications

Perforation and haemorrhage can in theory occur, but are most unlikely. The management of these complications will be described in Chapter 7.

Removal of less dense adhesions

Equipment

• Small-bore or microcolpohysteroscope, with scissors integral to the external sheath, or semi-rigid (Fig. 5.4).
• Paracervical block kit.
• An intra-uterine device.

Technique

Very fine adhesions can be disrupted easily by pressing upon them with the tip of the hysteroscope.

Thicker adhesions require more detailed attention. Two simple techniques can be used. Both require the administration of local anaesthesia. The surgeon must first identify the intra-uterine landmarks. Dissection may be necessary to unmask the tubal ostia.

The first technique, target abrasion, depends upon the properties of the microcolpohysteroscope. It will be noted that the tip is angled rather like a chisel. Using × 20 magnification an avascular area at one pole of the adhesion is identified. The tip of the hysteroscope is used like a chisel to make a 1 mm deep bite into this area. After each bite the area is observed to ensure that no false passages are being created. A series of such bites will free the adhesions. Target abrasion can be performed using carbon dioxide as the distension medium.

The second approach is to use scissors, either mounted on an integral sheath or introduced through a channel in the operating sheath, to divide the adhesions. Introduction of these instruments may require some cervical dilatation. Hyskon is an ideal distension medium.

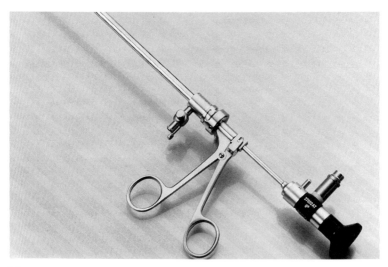

(a)

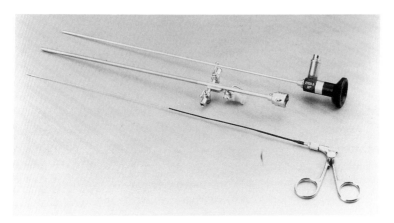

(b)

Fig. 5.4 Hysteroscope with: (a) rigid integral scissors; (b) semi-rigid scissors.

Follow-up

In order to prevent re-formation an intra-uterine device should be inserted when all but the filmiest adhesions have been divided. Regeneration of the endometrium is encouraged by prescribing an estrogen for 6 weeks and adding a progestational agent for the last 14 days. (Ethinylestradiol 100 mg plus medroxyprogesterone acetate 10 mg.) When the medication is discontinued, withdrawal bleeding will occur. An out-patient hysteroscopy is performed once the bleeding has subsided. The device is removed and any adhesions which may have re-formed will be soft and easily broken down.

Complications

It may prove impossible to complete the procedure. The more dense the adhesions, the more laterally situated, and the closer to the tubal ostia the greater the risk of perforation.

Methods of dealing with adhesions which cannot be removed simply, and with uterine perforation will be described in chapters 5–7.

Removal of non-embedded IUCDs

Equipment

- Basic equipment.
- Grasping forceps.
- Heavy duty grasping forceps.

Technique

The IUCD is visualized. It must clearly not be penetrating the uterine wall. Its position is noted. If the string is easily accessible it can be grasped with fine forceps (Fig. 5.5), the hysteroscope and forceps are withdrawn and the string will follow. If the device is normally situated and the patient wishes to continue to use this form of contraception, nothing further need be done. If she wishes to have it removed, the lightweight hysteroscopic forceps are removed and the

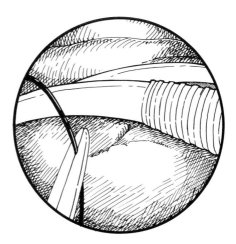

Fig. 5.5 'Lost IUCD'. The forceps are grasping the thread of the IUCD.

string seized with the heavy duty forceps. Removal proceeds. If the string is inaccessible, larger hysteroscopic forceps will be required with which to grasp the device itself. Once attached the forceps are withdrawn until the device is snug against the tip of the hystero-scope. All are withdrawn simultaneously. Incidentally, this technique has been used successfully in a female orangutan, albeit using general anaesthesia for the protection of the surgeon who was more apprehensive than the patient.

Follow-up

Follow-up will be directed by the patient's wishes. If the device has been left *in situ*, or if a new device was inserted immediately post-operatively, the patient should be examined following her next menstrual period to ensure that the strings are palpable. If the patient no longer wishes to use an IUCD her contraceptive needs must be met with an alternative method.

Complications

The complications are those of diagnostic hysteroscopy. Two situations can arise which warrant further discussion:
1 The embedded device. If the device has invaded the uterine wall no attempt should be made to remove it. Management of this situation will be described in Chapter 6.
2 The uterus is seen to be empty. If this is the case, a straight X-ray of the entire abdomen should be ordered. Translocated devices can lie anywhere within the abdominal cavity, including the sub-diaphragmatic area.

Tubal cannulation

Equipment

- Basic equipment.
- Tubal cannula.

Technique

No anaesthesia is required. The tubal ostium is visualized and the cannula passed. (This technique has little application.) Access to the tubes can be achieved more easily by radiographic or ultrasono-graphic guidance. In cases of suspected cornual obstruction, hysteroscopic cannulation and chromopertubation, or falloposcopy may occasionally be of value.

Follow-up

Follow-up will be dependent upon the indication for which tubal cannulation was performed.

Complications

The tube is a very delicate structure. Perforation can occur.

Tubal sterilization

The search continues for an effective, non-invasive, method of hysteroscopically directed tubal sterilization. The most promising is a nylon plug which is under investigation by Hamou and his colleagues. It has a coil at each end. The distal holds the device in place while the proximal, which remains in the uterine cavity, allows the device to be removed. Two devices are fitted into the 1.5 mm inserting catheter. The catheter contains a plunger which is used to insert the plugs.

Equipment

- Basic equipment.
- Plugs and introducer.

Technique

Hysteroscopy is performed and the right tubal ostium visualized. The introducer is fed along the operative channel until the tip can be seen (Fig. 5.6). The tip of the introducer is placed close to the ostium and the plunger advanced to insert the device to a depth of 1–2 cm. The procedure is repeated in the left tube.

Follow-up and complications

At this time the technique is experimental. In some patients violent cramps have been experienced at the time of fitting. Acute pelvic inflammatory disease has occurred. Expulsion has been noted at the time of follow-up hysteroscopy. Intra-uterine and ectopic pregnancies have been reported.

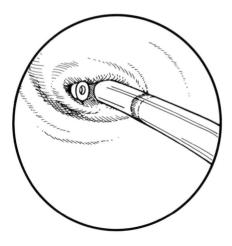

Fig. 5.6 Injection of silastic to occlude the fallopian tube.

Conclusions

With proper equipment and training a series of simple operative procedures can be carried out hysteroscopically in an out-patient department. They will require no or local anaesthesia only. It must be remembered that all tissues which have been removed must be submitted for histological evaluation. The complication rate for these procedures is extremely low.

6: Complex Operative Procedures

Introduction

Simple operative procedures were defined as those usually requiring no or local anaesthesia only. Complex operative procedures are performed with the patient under general anaesthesia. This is both because the procedures are inherently painful, and because the operating time is often in excess of 1 hour. To ask anyone to remain in the lithotomy position for such a long time while fully awake would be inhumane.

As techniques improve and operating times are steadily diminished, some or indeed most of these operations may well be carried out under local anaesthesia or a combination of local anaesthesia and parenterally administered narcoleptic agents.

Simple procedures are performed in out-patient facilities. The more complex usually require same day admission and post-operative overnight stay. Once again there is a shift towards same day discharge.

This chapter will discuss the principles of complex hysteroscopic surgery and then describe in detail the techniques of the individual operations.

Principles

Preparation of the surgeon

None of the procedures to be described in this chapter should be performed by any gynaecologist unless they:
• have completed the training described in Chapter 8;
• are fully able to perform any of the procedures by traditional methods;

- are thoroughly familiar with the complications, and their prevention;
- are fully capable of dealing with any complications which might arise.

Surgeons in training should ideally progress from the least to the most difficult operation, becoming more confident as they do so. This chapter has been structured so as to describe the complex operative procedures in this sequential fashion. Removal of heterotopic bone is not particularly difficult. It concludes the chapter simply because of the likelihood that few hysteroscopists will encounter this rare condition.

Finally it is incumbent upon any surgeon to make every reasonable endeavour to gain access to and be familiar with the patient's previous medical records.

Preparation of the patient

Patients should only undergo complex hysteroscopic procedures if they have:
- been deemed fit for general anaesthesia;
- been assured not to be at risk from fluid overload;
- been found not to be suffering from overt or potential acute pelvic inflammation;
- completed any necessary pre-operative investigations of their presenting symptom;
- if necessary, undergone diagnostic hysteroscopy and endometrial biopsy;
- completed any non-surgical management of their presenting complaint;
- taken the full course of any medications prescribed to facilitate their operation;
- given fully informed consent following discussion of the alternatives to surgery, and risks, complications and potential benefits of the proposed procedure.

Anaesthesia and positioning

General anaesthesia will be induced with the patient supine on the operating table. The choice of anaesthetic agents and the decision whether or not to intubate the patient belong in the realm of the anaesthetist. The anaesthetist must ensure that any monitoring leads are properly grounded. Burns can occur at the site of application of these monitoring devices when electrocautery is used. Once asleep the patient is placed in the lithotomy position. Both legs should be lifted simultaneously to avoid strain to the lumbar spine of the patient. The legs are placed in the lithotomy stirrups in a fashion which avoids exerting pressure on the major nerves of the leg. Before the table is broken or the lower half removed, the surgeon must ensure that the patient's hands are not at risk from moving parts of the table.

Once the table has been positioned to give access to the perineum, the patient is placed so that her buttocks protrude beyond the edge of the table. It may be necessary to depress the hysteroscope, and sufficient room should be left so that this manoeuvre can be performed.

The return electrode is applied. It must be remembered that any metal parts of the table which come into contact with the patient may act as return electrodes. Burns can occur at such sites. The surgeon must be sure that such risks are avoided. (Even if scissors or laser are the instruments to be used, instant availability of electrocautery may be invaluable if bleeding occurs.)

The perineum and vagina are cleansed with an antiseptic solution and the patient is draped. If prolonged operating time is anticipated a catch sheet, as used in urology, should be placed under the patient so that any distension medium which has leaked from the cervix or through the instruments can be collected and measured. A bimanual examination is performed and the size, and particularly position, of the uterus noted. The easiest method of perforation is to perform hysteroscopy in a patient who harbours an unsuspectedly retroverted uterus. For short procedures it is sufficient that the patient void immediately pre-operatively. For longer procedures in which large volumes of fluid may be used a Foley catheter should be inserted. The catheter is attached to a drainage bag so that intra- and post-operative urinary output can be measured accurately.

If concomitant laparoscopy is to be performed this is now undertaken and the initial pelvic survey performed. With the patient in the Trendelenburg position the small bowel is pushed from the pelvis into the upper abdomen by using the blunt probe. Even if laparoscopy is not performed, a degree of Trendelenburg position both prevents the weighted speculum from falling out and may encourage some of the small bowel to fall from the pelvis into the upper abdomen, and hence be less at risk should uterine perforation occur.

The weighted speculum is inserted, the cervix visualized and a tenaculum applied firmly. If cervical dilatation is required, as will almost invariably be the case, the surgeon proceeds to dilate the cervix to a size of dilator which is just smaller than the diameter of the external sheath of the hysteroscope. In this way a medium tight seal at the cervix can be ensured.

The surgery can now begin, it is worth restating that the surgeon must have confirmed, prior to induction of anaesthesia, that all the equipment is in working order.

The hysteroscope required to perform the specific operation is inserted with its camera attached. Most complex hysteroscopic surgery should be performed using the video monitor to display the uterine cavity. The speculum is removed. The surgeon may find it simpler to follow these steps while standing. Once the hysteroscope has been inserted the surgeon sits and the table is brought to a comfortable height.

The surgeon confirms that satisfactory uterine distension has occurred. The first step, as always, is to become orientated within the uterine cavity by identifying the tubal ostia. The lesion is evaluated and its limits defined. The surgery is completed. During this surgery constant attention must be paid to the intake and output of any fluid distension medium, and the surgeon appraised of any net deficit. If the deficit exceeds 1 l the operation must be completed as soon as possible. If it exceeds 2 l the operation must be abandoned.

Once the surgery has been completed a final uterine survey is made with the distension pressure at a low setting. This will reveal any bleeding vessels which may have been tamponaded by the higher intra-uterine pressure. Once satisfied that the uterus is dry, or that any further steps to ensure haemostasis (see later in this chapter) have been taken, the hysteroscope is removed

The weighted speculum is replaced and the tenaculum removed. The tenaculum puncture sites are inspected and confirmed to be dry. Neglect of this simple step results in more trips to the emergency department in the middle of the night than any of the other possible complications of hysteroscopy. The speculum is removed. If a coloured antiseptic solution has been used it is a simple courtesy to wash it off before taking the patient out of the lithotomy position. Once again ensuring that all parts of the patient are clear of the working parts of the table, the lower end is restored to its position. The table is taken from the Trendelenburg position. The legs are removed from the lithotomy stirrups as they were placed there to avoid strain to the lumbar spine.

Before leaving the operating room to complete the documentation of the procedure, the surgeon once again compares the amount of fluid taken in with the total amount in the suction apparatus, the catch sheet and the urinary drainage bag.

These principles apply irrespective of the instrument used. Some aspects of technique vary dependent upon whether:

1 scissors,
2 the resectoscope or
3 the laser

are used. These will now be discussed.

Scissors

Scissors for use in complex hysteroscopic surgical procedures may be:

• integral to the sheath;
• passed through an operating channel. In this case rigid as opposed to semi-rigid or flexible instruments are preferable.

They can be used to deal with septa or dense adhesions. These are usually bloodless procedures. Since this is the case, integral scissors can be used with carbon dioxide. These instruments are of small enough diameter that cervical dilatation is not required. Insertion of the sheath to accommodate rigid scissors will require cervical dilatation. As this can cause bleeding, use of a liquid medium is preferable. Although electroconductivity should not be a consideration in the selection of the medium, thus suggesting saline or high molecular weight dextran, any complex hysteroscopic procedure may cause intra-uterine haemorrhage. Electrocautery may be required to control this bleeding at which time the nature of the fluid does become important. Use of sorbitol or glycine as the primary distension medium of choice resolves this difficulty. Never use an electrolytic solution with electrocautery.

The technique of the use of scissors, irrespective of the lesion being treated involves the following steps:

• no attempt should be made to divide any structure until it has been completely identified;
• the tips of the scissors must be kept under constant observation;
• it is preferable where possible to take full-sized bites with the blades;
• if progress is difficult, small bites may be taken to free lesions which are obstructing the field of view.

The resectoscope

The construction of this instrument has been described in Chapter 2. It can be used to excise large polyps and submucous fibroids, divide uterine septa, and destroy the endometrium. The technique of its use, irrespective of the lesion being treated, involves the following steps:

• assembling and testing;
• use of a fluid (sorbitol or glycine);
• use of a pump delivery sytem;
• use of a suction system attached to the outflow stopcock;
• use of a compatible electrosurgical generator. The wattage setting and current mode (cutting, coagulating or blended) will depend upon the procedure to be performed;
• the cervix must be dilated to a size just smaller than the external sheath;
• the external sheath, which is equipped with an obturator, is inserted;
• the obturator is withdrawn and the remainder of the resectoscope inserted in its place;
• fluid flow is commenced with the outflow stopcock shut until the uterus is satisfactorily distended;
• the outflow stopcock, connected to a suction system set at 30 mmHg, is opened;
• inflow pressures should be maintained at about 80–100 mmHg;
• the surgeon becomes orientated by identifying the tubal ostia;
• the nature and extent of the lesion is assessed;
• no current is ever passed unless the active element can be kept under direct vision;
• strokes with the active element must always be made from the fundus towards the cervix. Strokes made in the opposite direction greatly increase the risk of uterine perforation;
• the cornua are the thinnest (6 mm) and hence most easily perforated areas of the uterine wall;
• the active element can be advanced and retracted by pressure on the proximal grip, by moving the entire resectoscope forwards and backwards, or by a combination of the two;
• debris can be removed by withdrawing the resectoscope from the external sheath and allowing the distension medium to flow out carrying the debris with it, or with polyp forceps;
• on each occasion that this step is performed time must be allowed to elapse, once the resectoscope has been replaced, for the uterus to redistend. Distension is absolutely necessary to maintain an adequate visual field. Sudden loss of the view means that distension has been lost. This can occur if an inflow stopcock has been closed inadvertently, the fluid containing bag is empty, or uterine perforation has occurred.

The laser

The laser hysteroscope is similar to the resectoscope. It does not have the working element, nor does it have as many sheaths. It is a three channel instrument, inflow, outflow and laser channel. Only the Nd : YAG laser is suitable for hysteroscopic surgery. It can be used with saline as the distension medium. Essentially the same steps as those described for the resectoscope are followed. Use of the laser for specific procedures will be discussed later.

The individual operations

More complex procedures carried out hysteroscopically include:
- combined laparoscopy and hysteroscopy;
- excision of large or multiple polyps;
- excision of septa;
- excision of fibroids;
- endometrial ablation or resection;
- excision of extensive adhesions;
- removal of heterotopic bone.

These will now be described.

Combined laparoscopy and hysteroscopy

Indications

Laparoscopy and hysteroscopy may be carried out together:
1 to monitor complex hysteroscopic surgery if there is a risk of uterine perforation;
2 as part of the investigation of infertility;
3 as part of the investigation of habitual abortion;
4 to remove embedded IUCDs.

Pre-operative work-up

1 Routine as described earlier and in Chapter 4.
2 Specific as indicated by the presenting symptom:
  - To monitor complex hysteroscopic surgery — this will be described in the following sections.
  - Investigation of infertility. Laparoscopy may be combined with hysteroscopy in these patients if the HSG has identified an intra-uterine lesion or proximal tubal occlusion.
  - If the complaint is one of habitual abortion then when the timing

is right to evaluate the uterine cavity, the accuracy and simplicity of out-patient hysteroscopy suggest that this investigation can replace HSG. If a uterine malformation can be so identified, laparoscopy will be required to evaluate the external configuration of the uterus so that septate malformations can be differentiated from bicornuate malformations

- The embedded IUCD — the situation of the device will have been determined by out-patient hysteroscopy. Those that are partly within the uterine cavity but partly embedded in the uterine wall will require combined laparoscopy and hysteroscopy to be performed.

Equipment

In the investigation of infertility:
- small bore diagnostic hysteroscope using carbon dioxide;
- operative hysteroscopic equipment on stand-by so that if the lesion is amenable to hysteroscopic surgery it can be performed immediately;
- chromopertubation cannula and solution;
- tubal cannula.

In the management of habitual abortion:
- if fibroids are to be treated the resectoscope should be available;
- septa can be dealt with using scissors or the resectoscope.

The embedded IUCD:
- hysteroscope with operative sheath capable of carrying strong forceps.

Technique

To monitor complex hysteroscopic surgery. When complex hysteroscopic surgery is to be monitored the laparoscope is inserted in the usual fashion. A probe is introduced in the mid-line, and with the patient in the Trendelenburg position the bowel is pushed from the pelvis. Once the hysteroscopic surgery has commenced the light of the laparoscope is extinguished. Imminent uterine perforation is signalled if the transillumination of the uterine wall becomes very bright. If perforation occurs the hysteroscopy is discontinued, the laparoscope is reilluminated and any damage to the uterus or intra-pelvic structures is assessed.

The transillumination of the uterus can also be used as an indication of satisfactory division of a septum or adhesiolysis. Once the hysteroscopic surgeon believes the uterine cavity to have been returned to normality, the telescope is placed in one cornu and slowly swept across the fundus to the other cornu. If the laparoscopist observes consistency in the intensity of the transillumination it is reasonable to assume that indeed the surgery has been completed satisfactorily. Monitoring for imminent perforation and assessment of the surgical result can also be carried out ultrasonographically.

Investigation of the infertile patient. Diagnostic hysteroscopy is performed first. The findings are noted and the hysteroscope removed. If small lesions had been identified hysteroscopically they can be dealt with as described in Chapter 5. The chromopertubation cannula is locked to the tenaculum. If the order of these steps is reversed, cervical bleeding caused by the cannula and the dye solution may hinder hysteroscopic visualization. The laparoscopy and chromopertubation are carried out in a routine fashion. The presence or absence of cornual obstruction can be assessed by introducing a soft catheter into the tubal ostium using hysteroscopic guidance (Fig. 6.1). The results of hydropertubation through this catheter can be observed laparoscopically. More significant lesions (myomata, septa, dense adhesions) will be treated as will be described later in this chapter. This surgery can be monitored laparoscopically. Once the surgery has been completed both instruments are removed as described previously.

Habitual abortion. If a uterine malformation has been identified at the time of diagnostic hysteroscopy, then laparoscopy is performed first. If there is evidence of a bicornuate deformity, hysteroscopy is not indicated. The patient may wish to undergo laparotomy and formal

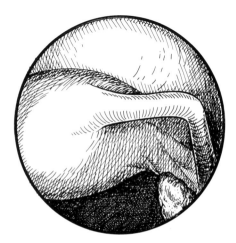

Fig. 6.1 Laparoscopic view of the tube with a cannula in the lumen of the isthmus.

uterine reunification. If the uterus appears to be of normal external configuration the diagnosis of a septate uterus is confirmed. This can be dealt with immediately by hysteroscopic means under laparoscopic monitoring.

The embedded IUCD. Laparoscopy is performed first. If the device is predominantly in the abdominal cavity, or if of a T-shaped configuration and the cross piece of the T is extra-uterine, attempts should be made to remove it with laparoscopic grasping forceps (Fig. 6.2). If removal is successful the uterine surface is inspected to evaluate the degree of bleeding.

If the device is adherent to bowel or omentum, as is often the case with those bearing copper, it also must be removed from above. It may be necessary first to dissect off the adherent structures (Fig. 6.3). If removal from above is successful, hysteroscopy is not required.

If at the time of laparoscopy it is judged that the IUCD is predominantly within the myometrium and uterine cavity, and it is completely free from, or has laparoscopically been freed from, adherence to adjacent structures, hysteroscopy should be performed (Fig. 6.4). An operative hysteroscope should be used with heavy grasping forceps. Because there may be significant loss of uterine integrity when the device has been removed, neither carbon dioxide nor high molecular weight dextran should be used. The former carries a theoretical risk of gas embolism, the latter of anaphylaxis if sufficient quantities gain access to the circulation.

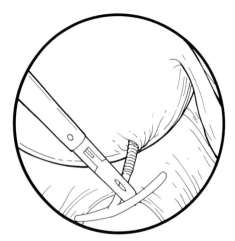

Fig. 6.2 Laparascopic view of penetrating intra-uterine device being removed with forceps.

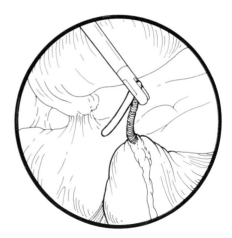

Fig. 6.3 Penetrating IUCD buried in omentum. Laparascopic view of device being extracted.

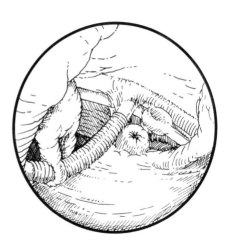

Fig. 6.4 IUCD with the endometrium growing over it and the tips buried.

Once the hysteroscope is inserted and the surgeon has identified the uterine landmarks, the grasping forceps are inserted. It is usually futile to try pulling on the string. It usually snaps. The device should be grasped firmly by any accessible part. Slow firm traction is exerted. The surgeon should be prepared for it to come loose suddenly and may wish to reduce the tractive force as the IUCD gradually comes free. Once the device is free the defect in the uterine wall is inspected to ensure that there is no heavy bleeding. Device, forceps and hysteroscope are removed simultaneously.

The uterine surface is inspected laparoscopically to ensure that there is no major bleeding. If there is a considerable amount of distension fluid in the pelvis it can be aspirated through a laparoscopically guided catheter.

Large or multiple polyps

Pre-operative work-up

- Routine as described earlier and in Chapter 4.
- Specific, prior diagnostic hysteroscopy and endometrial biopsy.

Equipment

- Diagnostic hysteroscope.
- Operating hysteroscope plus grasping forceps.
- Resectoscope.
- Fluid medium and delivery system.
- Dilatation and curettage set.
- Nd : YAG laser.

Technique

The previous diagnostic hysteroscopy will have determined whether there is a single large polyp or multiple polyps. Multiple polyposis is difficult to deal with hysteroscopically. Blind curettage tends to fail to remove all of the lesions. Directed curettage gives the best results. The cervix is dilated and a diagnostic hysteroscope using a fluid medium is inserted. The number and sites of the polyps are identified. The hysteroscope is removed and curettage performed, directing the curette sequentially to the known locations of the lesions. Once the surgeon believes that all of the polyps have been removed the diagnostic hysteroscope is reintroduced. The curettage will have produced bleeding which would obscure the view if carbon dioxide were used. An immiscible fluid (high molecular weight dextran) or a continuous flow hysteroscope will overcome this difficulty. If the uterus is judged to be empty the procedure is discontinued. If residual lesions are noted it may be possible to avulse them with the hysteroscopically directed grasping forceps, or it may be necessary to repeat the steps of directed curettage. This procedure does not require laparoscopic monitoring. It is also possible to remove multiple small polyps with the resectoscope loop or the laser. Large (greater than 2 cm) single polyps will be treated using the resectoscope or Nd : YAG laser in the manner to be described for submucous fibroids.

Excision of septa

Pre-operative work-up

- Routine, as described earlier and in Chapter 4.
- Specific, diagnostic hysteroscopy.

Equipment

- Resectoscope, or operating hysteroscope plus scissors, or Nd : YAG laser.
- Fluid distension medium and delivery system.
- Laparoscopic or ultrasound monitoring.

Technique

Monitoring to prevent uterine perforation and to assess the thickness of the uterine fundus is desirable. Either a laparoscopy is performed or transabdominal ultrasound scanning is begun. The cervix is dilated and the hysteroscope or resectoscope inserted. Both hemi-uterine cavities are explored and the tubal ostia identified.

The length and breadth of the septum is evaluated. The objective of the operation is to create a uterine cavity which is normal in both shape and volume. This will be achieved by cutting the septum transversely (sagitally) in a line joining the two tubal ostia, which are used as the essential landmarks towards the end of the incision. It is unnecessary to excise the septum because, when it is divided, the anterior and posterior uterine walls spring apart creating the new cavity with the remains of the septum showing as a triangular area bereft of endometrium with its base the line between the two tubal ostia. It must be remembered that the normal fundus is convex. Attempts to achieve flatness of the fundus may lead to haemorrhage and perforation.

The techniques of incision differ depending upon the instrument used. When the resectoscope is used to excise a septum the loop is replaced with a cutting blade. The blade is set at a right angle to the shaft of the element. It is 7 mm long and can be used to measure the distance from the tubal orifice. This adds a degree of safety to the procedure. The generator is set at a blended current with 80 watts of cutting and 40 watts of coagulation. The resectoscope is placed so that the blade is in contact with the edge of the septum which is closer to the cervix (Fig. 6.5a). It is rotated so that the tip of the cutting blade faces one hemi-cavity and the heel of the blade is used

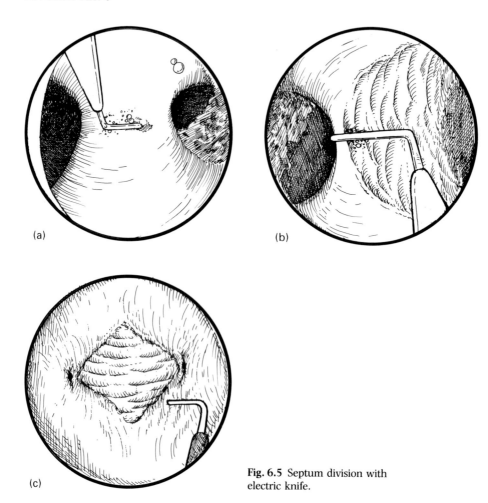

(a)

(b)

(c)

Fig. 6.5 Septum division with electric knife.

to make the incision. The current is applied in very short bursts of about 1–2 seconds. Cutting proceeds at a rate of about 1–2 mm per application. When some progress has been made on one side the instrument is rotated through 180° and the process repeated (Fig. 6.5b). The incision proceeds gradually in this alternating fashion until the desired appearance of the cavity is noted. If the base of the septum extends to the cornua it is possible to incise it to within a few millimetres of the ostia by using the knife as a ruler. The incision should be halted about 4 mm from the margin of the ostium (Fig. 6.5c).

If a hysteroscope which has scissors as part of the external sheath is used, carbon dioxide can be an effective distension medium. However, great care must be taken to avoid causing bleeding during passage of the cervix, otherwise bubbles will occlude the field of view.

If rigid scissors are passed through an operating sheath, Hyskon is the medium of choice. Modern operating hysteroscopes have continuous flow capability. Hyskon is not miscible with blood, and because of its high viscosity much smaller volumes are required. The blades of the scissors are applied to the cervical end of the septum. Whereas very small bites are taken with the resectoscope, initially the full bite of the scissors is used (Fig. 6.6). As the fundus is approached the bite size is reduced. A small amount of bleeding will occur when the scissors leave the septum and begin to incise healthy myometrium. At this point dissection should be discontinued.

The Nd : YAG laser must be used with a fluid medium. The power is set at 60–100 watts. A sapphire tip is fitted to the laser fibre. The fibre is used in the contact mode and the septum is progressively incised from its cervical end.

If the septum is complete, that is extending to the external os, the cervical portion should be divided with scissors. Hysteroscopic division of the uterine septum is performed 2 months later.

Because of the risk of post-operative adhesion formation it has been recommended that a large IUCD be inserted, and that the patient take high doses of ovarian steriods. We have not found this to be necessary.

Large or multiple fibroids

Fibroids may require to be removed in patients complaining of infertility, habitual abortion or heavy vaginal bleeding. Enormous advances have been made in the hysteroscopic management of fibroids. Operations which were considered impossible a few years ago are now becoming commonplace. There is no longer only one

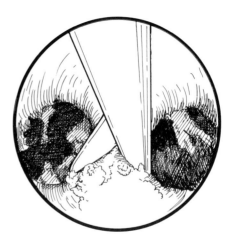

Fig. 6.6 Resection of septum with scissors.

approach. Single fibroids can be dealt with hysteroscopically by a one step removal, or with medical suppression followed by a one step removal. Larger lesions may require suppression and removal in two steps. Multiple lesions should be removed individually in a series of operations. Both the size and the ratio between that part of the tumour in the cavity and that part in the myometrium must be considered. Based upon these considerations a classification has been devised.

Classification

Table 6.1 demonstrates the management as dictated by tumour size and cavity intra-mural ratio (CIR).

In addition to these considerations the anatomical position within the uterus will influence the degree of difficulty of the surgery and the technique. Lesions of the lateral, anterior and posterior walls are equally accessible to laser and electrosurgery. Lesions of the fundus, especially if deeply sited, are more amenable to laser treatment (Fig. 6.7). These positional considerations do not influence the need for pre-treatment. Irrespective of their size those fibroids which are close to or causing obstruction of the tube should be suppressed before removal. Finally, if there are multiple lesions each is assessed on its individual characteristics. The criteria for single lesions are applied to the management decision. However they should be removed one at a time at several sessions, separated by 2-month intervals if they are on opposite walls of the uterus. If such lesions were to be removed simultaneously the risk of adhesion formation would be prohibitive.

Pre-operative work-up

- Routine as described earlier.
- Assessment of the size, relationships, and number of the fibroids.

Table 6.1 Treatment regime as determined by tumour diameter and CIR

CIR	Tumour diameter (cm)		
	< 2.5	2.5–5.0	> 5.0
> 75	One step	One step	Suppression + one step
75–50	One step	Suppression + one step	Suppression + one step
< 50	Suppression + one step	Suppression + one or two steps	Suppression + two steps

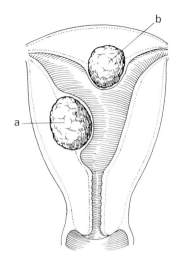

Fig. 6.7 A lateral wall fibroid (a) can be removed easily with a resectoscope loop. It is more difficult to apply the loop to a fundal fibroid (b).

The bimanual examination is of critical importance. If the uterus is larger than the size of a 14 week pregnancy, hysteroscopic surgery is contra-indicated. If the uterus is of normal size and the presence of a submucous fibroid is suspected, diagnostic hysteroscopy should be performed. A concurrent endometrial biopsy should be routine in all cases as frequently there will be evidence of endometrial hyperplasia in the vicinity of the tumour.

When the uterine size is between normality and 14 weeks it is probable that there will be multiple or intra-mural fibroids. Trans-vaginal ultrasonography will identify the position and number of the lesions. The maximum diameter of each should be measured. Diagnostic hysteroscopy will delineate the nature of the uterine cavity.

Hysterosalpingography can be performed as a routine in all patients with evidence of fibroids, or selectively in infertile patients in whom lesions in close proximity with the intra-mural segment of the tube have been identified.

This information will allow a logical treatment protocol to be developed for each individual patient.

Equipment

• Resectoscope with cutting loop, knife and roller ball, or operative hysteroscope and Nd : YAG laser.
• Fluid distension medium and pump.

Although it is not necessary to monitor hysteroscopic myomectomy the laparoscopic equipment should be instantly available. Although rare, perforations can occur and immediate evaluation of the abdominal contents will be indicated.

Technique

Medical suppression. The need to suppress certain tumours has been mentioned earlier. This approach is implemented in those circumstances in which it is necessary to reduce the size, volume and vascularity of the intra-mural portion. Progestational agents, danazol and gonadotrophin releasing hormone agonists (GnRHA) may reduce the volume of fibroids by 30–60%. It should be remembered that the size of the uterine cavity may also be reduced so that there is little net gain in the available working space. Occasionally, suppression may be so effective that the tumour virtually disappears. Although it will regain its orginal size in about 3 months, in cases of infertility this may provide a window during which conception may occur. Conversely some tumours, particularly those within the cavity, may not have responded. All patients who have taken suppressive therapy should be reassessed ultrasonographically and if appropriate by hysterosalpingography.

Both progestational agents and danazol may give rise to a number of side-effects which adversely affect patient compliance. If a depot GnRHA is given the surgeon can be confident that the medication is exerting its desired action. Our preference is to use goserelin depot in a dose of 3.6 mg given by deep subcutaneous injection.

Specific procedures

The degree to which the tumour protrudes into the uterine cavity will indicate the surgical approach (Fig. 6.8). The need to use suppressive therapy is predicated by tumour size. The resectoscope or laser can be used.

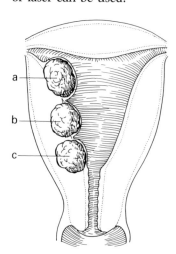

Fig. 6.8 (a) Fibroid more than 50% intracavity; (b) fibroid 50% intracavity; (c) fibroid less than 50% intracavity.

Lesions which are more than 75% intra-cavity (submucous). Hystero-scopic removal of these lesions is relatively simple provided that they are less than 2.5 cm in diameter. The surgeon in training should first master the technique of dealing with these small fibroids before attempting to operate on larger intra-cavity lesions. The surgeon should be competent in the management of intra-cavity fibroids before attempting to remove intra-mural fibroids, or to perform endometrial destruction.

Submucous fibroids may be removed without prior suppression unless they are greater than 5 cm in diameter. Goserelin is given 4 weeks pre-operatively to patients who harbour larger lesions. Pro-vided these fibroids shrink to 5 cm or less they can then be treated like originally smaller lesions.

Submucous fibroids may be sessile or pedunculated.

Electrosurgery of sessile fibroids. The current is set in a blended mode with 80 watts of both coagulating and cutting current. The loop is advanced to the distal extremity of the tumour and an incision made in the surface (Fig. 6.9). The direction of cutting is from the fundus towards the cervix.

The excised tissue can either be removed through the external sheath or left to float freely. Successive slices are taken until the uterine wall is flat. If floating debris becomes troublesome and obscures the view the resectoscope is removed and the pieces extracted with ring forceps or a blunt curette. The junction between the pale fibrous tissues of the myoma and the striated myometrium is easily recognized and indicates that excision is complete.

Laser surgery of sessile fibroids. The power is set at 60–100 watts. If the laser is defocused it can be used to vaporize the lesion commenc-ing with the pole which is closest to the cervix and moving towards the fundus (Fig. 6.10). (While this is safe with the laser, electrocau-tery must never be used in this direction.) Alternatively the laser fibre can be used to dissect the tumour from its bed by cutting in the plane of cleavage (Fig. 6.11). Once the tumour is lying freely within the cavity it can be removed with ring forceps. If difficulty is experienced with this removal the fibroid can be left in the cavity as it will be expelled spontaneously within the next few days.

Surgery of pedunculated fibroids. A narrow pedicle can be divided with the electric knife, resection loop or laser (Fig. 6.12). Once free the tumour can be removed with ring forceps or left to be passed. If it is difficult to gain access to the pedicle, the fibroid can be removed with

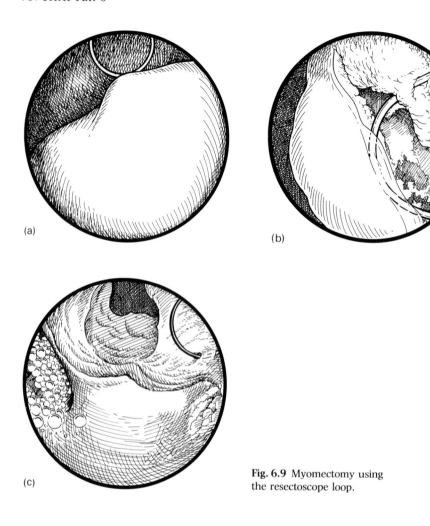

(a)

(b)

(c)

Fig. 6.9 Myomectomy using the resectoscope loop.

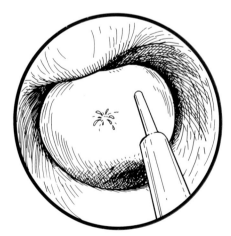

Fig. 6.10 Vaporization of submucous fibroid using Nd : YAG laser.

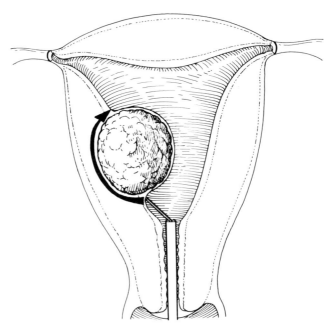

Fig. 6.11 Nd : YAG laser dissection commences at the lower pole of the fibroid and proceeds distally.

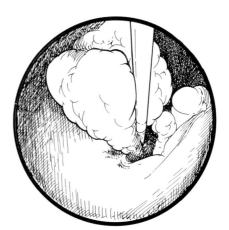

Fig.6.12 Nd : YAG laser vaporizing the pedicle of a sessile submucous fibroid.

the resectoscope or vaporized with the laser. One disadvantage of laser vaporization or leaving the severed tumour in the uterine cavity is that no tissue will be available for histological evaluation.

Lesions which are 75–50% intra-cavity. Any such fibroid which is greater than 2.5 cm in diameter should be medically suppressed prior to surgery, using the same regime as described for submucous lesions. The technique of electrical excision is similar to that used to remove sessile submucous myomata up to the point when the resection reaches the level of the surrounding myometrium. Although the mechanism is unclear, the intra-mural portion will be spontaneously extruded into the cavity. Resection of this extruded tissue continues until normal myometrium is reached. This approach is simpler than dissecting the fibroid with the laser.

Lesions which are less than 50% intra-cavity. Hysteroscopic removal of such lesions is difficult and should not be undertaken by any but the most experienced surgeons. In all cases 2 months suppressive therapy should be given and if the lesion fails to shrink to a size of 5 cm or less, hysteroscopic surgery is contra-indicated. Small lesions of less than 2.5 cm are dealt with in a fashion similar to that just described. Two steps will be required for larger lesions. The first step proceeds as above, during which more and more of the fibroid is extruded into the cavity. A time will be reached when it will be felt prudent to stop because of the danger of bleeding or perforation. Myolysis is now performed by devitalizing the remaining tumour using electrical or laser energy. If the resectoscope is used, the loop is replaced with the knife and multiple holes are made in the residual tumour to a depth of 5 mm.

The surgery is now discontinued and suppressive therapy continued for another 2 months. During this time the devitalized fibroid will shrink, become avascular, pedunculated and submucous in position. Hysteroscopic removal is now easily performed as previously described.

Remarkably the myometrium which was compressed by the fibroid will have returned to its normal thickness. This operation does not leave the residual weakness in the uterine wall which was associated with conventional myomectomy.

If multiple, excisable lesions exist, those of one wall should be dealt with first. Those of the contra-lateral wall should be resected 2–3 months later. Simultaneous resection at two opposing surfaces carries an unacceptable risk of adhesion formation.

Gaining access to fundal fibroids with the resectoscope is difficult. They should be suppressed. It may be necessary to bend the loop to an angle of 135° from its supporting posts. If this step is taken the surgeon must ensure that the loop is always within the visual field. It may be necessary to perform the myomectomy as a two or even three stage procedure. Laser is easier and safer in these situations as the technique is the same as for lateral wall fibroids.

If the myomectomy has been performed for a woman who has completed her family and is suffering from menorrhagia it may be advisable to perform an endometrial ablation at the same time.

Endometrial ablation or resection

Endometrial ablation or resection is performed for the woman who has completed childbearing and who suffers from dysfunctional uterine bleeding of sufficient severity to warrant hysterectomy.

Ablation or resection is technically more difficult and unlikely to be successful if the uterine cavity is deeper than 12 cm.

Pre-operative work-up

- Routine as described earlier in this chapter.
- Confirmation that major risks from fluid overload are not present.
- Completion of unsuccessful non-surgical alternative treatment.
- Assessment of the depth and configuration of the uterine cavity by either hysteroscopy or transvaginal ultrasound.
- Endometrial biopsy. The procedure is contra-indicated if there is evidence of adenomatous hyperplasia, carcinoma *in situ*, or invasive carcinoma.
- Endometrial suppression for 1–2 months.

Danazol 600 mg daily may be given for 4–6 weeks pre-operatively. The occurrence of side-effects may affect patient compliance, so it is probably preferable to use GnRHA. The goserelin depot of 3.6 mg should be given at the start of a menstrual period and repeated 4 weeks later. The operation is scheduled for 5 weeks after the initial injection. This ensures adequate down regulation of the pituitary both pre- and post-operatively.

Equipment

Destruction of the endometrium can be effected by:
1 ablation using a roller electrode;
2 resection using a resectoscope loop;
3 a combination of 1 and 2; or
4 the Nd : YAG laser;
Instruments for laparoscopy should be available.

The equipment required for 1, 2 and 3 is the resectoscope and for 4 an Nd : YAG laser and a hysteroscope with a channel equipped to carry the laser fibre. The distal end of the fibre may be left bare or may be equipped with a sapphire tip.

Tubal occlusion does not prevent fluid absorption. Although the risk is low, conception could occur following ablation. Patients should at least be offered the opportunity to be sterilized at the time of surgery. If they concur, laparoscopy is performed first and the bowel pushed from the pelvis, then the sterilization is carried out and the laparoscope left *in situ* to monitor the intra-uterine surgery. The laparoscope should be on standby in case uterine perforation occurs.

Technique

Using electrical energy. The use of the roller ball is simplest. Resection may be somewhat more effective. A combination of both is probably the optimum technique.

In all cases the cervix is dilated, the resectoscope inserted and the landmarks are identified. If the ball electrode is to be used the current is set in a blended mode with 100 watts of cutting and 50 watts of coagulating current. The cornual regions are dealt with first. The ball is rolled over the endometrium at a rate of about 10–14 mm/second from the tubo-cornual junction in a radial, overlapping fashion. The length of each stroke is about 1 cm. Current is only applied as the ball travels from the fundus towards the cervix. The fundus itself is dealt with. This involves rotating the resectoscope through an angle of 90°. Sequential overlapping strokes are taken along the entire anterior, lateral and posterior uterine walls from the fundus to the level of the internal os. The technique is exactly that of roller-painting a ceiling. It is advisable to apply two and sometimes three 'coats' of electrical paint to ensure total ablation.

If resection is to be performed the current is set in the blended mode. The cornua are dealt with first. The sequence of destruction is as follows. The fundus is first resected in a series of short transverse strokes (Fig. 6.13). The groove thus created acts as a guide for the

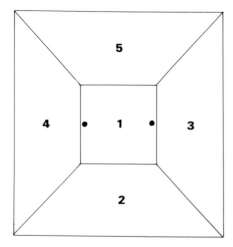

Fig. 6.13 In resection the fundus is treated first, followed by the posterior, lateral, and finally the anterior walls.

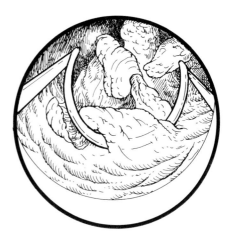

Fig. 6.14 The excised
endometrial strips accumulate
in the uterine fundus.

longitudinal incisions in the posterior wall. The first posterior incision is made in the mid-line. The full depth of the loop (4 mm)
should be used. In this way the entire thickness of the pink spongy
endometrium can be differentiated from the firm striated myometrium. The length of travel of the loop is 2.5 cm so each incision
will remove a strip of tissue of this length. A series of similar incisions
are made in a systematic manner to remove the endometrium of the
posterior and lateral walls of the fundus. Finally the endometrium of
the anterior fundal wall is resected. The initial removal of the
posterior tissues creates a convenient receptacle for the excised strips
of endometrium (Fig. 6.14). Once the full circumference of the
fundus has been treated the resectoscope is withdrawn for 2 cm and
the process repeated until the internal os has been reached. This is
recognized by the thinning of the endometrium which at this level is
paler. Another landmark is that the os can be seen in its entirety in
one visual field.

When the procedure has been completed the resectoscope is
removed, and the accumulated debris evacuated with ring forceps or
a curette. The resectoscope is reinserted and the uterus inspected to
ensure that no islands of endometrium have been missed and that
there is no bleeding (Fig. 6.15). To recognize bleeding reduce the
pressure of the distension medium. Small vessels can be spot
coagulated.

Many surgeons use a combination of both electrodes. Access to the
cornual regions and fundus is more easily achieved with the roller
electrode. The endometrium of the uterine cavity is then resected
with the loop. The ball is replaced. Bleeding points are coagulated
and the ridges between the resection incisions are treated with the
rollerball (Fig. 6.16).

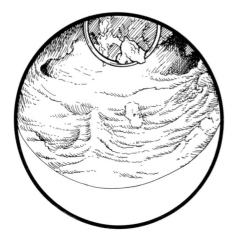

Fig. 6.15 Resection of posterior wall endometrium with resectoscope loop is almost complete.

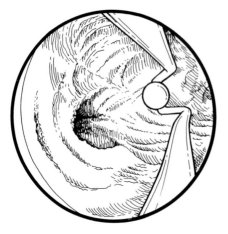

Fig. 6.16 The roller ball is used to coagulate the ridges and to treat the endometrium at the tubal insertion.

Using the Nd : YAG laser. The cervix is dilated and the operating hysteroscope inserted. A liquid distension medium is used. The laser is set at a wattage between 50 and 75. There are two techniques for applying the laser energy to the endometrial cavity, the touch and the non-touch. The touch technique is accomplished by allowing the quartz fibre to be in contact with the endometrium during the application of the laser energy. Yellow–brown furrows which are readily visible are created in the endometrium. The endometrium and, presumably, the superficial areas of myometrium, are actually vaporized as the quartz fibre cuts into tissue.

In the non-touch technique, the end of the fibre is brought as near to the lining of the uterus as possible without touching it (Fig. 6.17). The fibre is also directed as perpendicularly as possible to the uterine wall to decrease the amount of reflection and increase absorption.

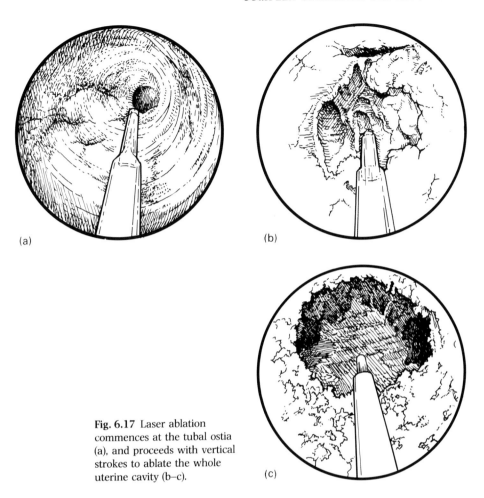

Fig. 6.17 Laser ablation commences at the tubal ostia (a), and proceeds with vertical strokes to ablate the whole uterine cavity (b–c).

The endometrium turns white and swells as it is coagulated but, unfortunately, this change is a less clear-cut endpoint than that seen in the touch technique. Occasionally, heat builds up beneath the surface causing small subendometrial explosions which will detach the endometrium.

A systematic approach in the uterine cavity is needed to minimize the chances of 'skipping' areas (Fig. 6.18). As in resection, ablation starts at the cornual and fundal areas, always using short, 5–10 second bursts of laser energy. The anterior wall is then ablated down to the internal os because bubbles and debris collect here and obscure the view. The lateral and finally, posterior walls are treated.

Unlike the bladder, the uterine cavity is small and it is difficult to apply the laser beam perpendicularly to the lower uterine segment even with the help of a deflecting arm. Thus, this area is difficult to treat using the non-touch technique. In the touch technique, the

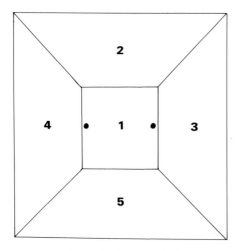

Fig. 6.18 In laser ablation the fundus is treated first, followed by the anterior, lateral, and finally the posterior walls.

fibre can simply be 'dragged' along the wall, thus some operators will often combine these two methods.

If the laser is used under direct vision, a special filter is required to be affixed to the eyepiece of the endoscope to protect the operator's eyes. This filter may wash out the contrasting colours of the uterine cavity. A high resolution video camera to display the image on a monitor as a means of retaining colour discrimination and protecting operating room personnel should be used.

Excision of extensive adhesions

Pre-operative work-up

- Routine as described earlier in this chapter.
- HSG.
- Diagnostic hysteroscopy.

Equipment

- Resectoscope, or Nd : YAG laser, or operating hysteroscope and scissors.
- Instruments for laparoscopy.
- IUCD.

Technique

This can be the most difficult hysteroscopic surgical procedure. Laparoscopic monitoring is recommended and the set-up is available for laparotomy if perforation should occur.

The cervix is dilated and the hysteroscope of choice inserted. The adhesions can be divided by the electric knife (set at 80 watts of cutting current), the laser (set at 75 watts) or scissors. Orientation is usually difficult as the adhesions often obscure the ostia (Fig. 6.19a). The resection begins laterally. In this situation all cutting must be directed towards the fundus. For this reason many surgeons prefer to use scissors at least in the initial part of the dissection (Fig. 6.19b). Perforation with scissors is less likely to produce the degree of intra-abdominal damage than that caused by electrical or laser energy. Dissection proceeds until the ostium can be identified (Fig. 6.19c). Further dissection is carried out laterally until the other ostium is visible and the surgeon is satisfied that the uterine cavity

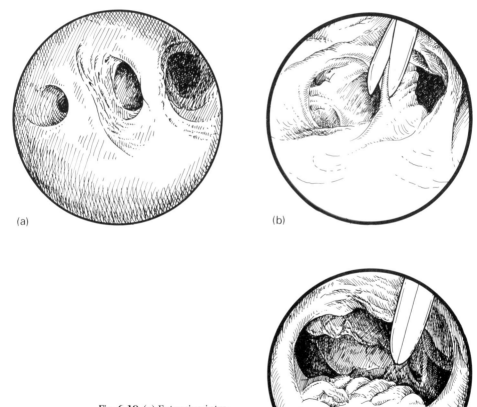

(a)

(b)

Fig. 6.19 (a) Extensive intra-uterine synechiae;
(b) division of the synechiae with scissors; (c) operation almost complete with the uterine cavity visible.

(c)

has a relatively normal configuration. The hysteroscope is removed and the IUCD inserted.

Removal of heterotopic bone

Pre-operative work-up

- General work-up.
- Diagnostic hysteroscopy.

Equipment

- Operative hysteroscope.
- Grasping forceps.
- Ball point electrode for use with the operating hysteroscope.

Technique

Cervical dilatation is not usually required. A small bore hysteroscope is inserted using carbon dioxide as the distension medium. The landmarks are identified and the bony tissue evaluated. The distal extremity of the hysteroscope can be used to dislodge the bony fragments. The grasping forceps are inserted. Any fragments which were not freed with the tip of the hysteroscope can be grasped and traction exerted. Once all the bony elements are free within the cavity, one is grasped and hysteroscope, forceps and fragment removed en bloc. This procedure may need to be repeated several times. Fragments 6 mm or more in size may need to be morcellated with the grasping forceps prior to removal. Once the uterine cavity is empty the hysteroscope is reinserted. The current is set at 15 watts of pure coagulating power, the electrode passed and the regions from which the bone was removed are lightly coagulated.

Conclusions

Surgical correction of some uterine lesions which once required major abdominal intervention can now be performed hysteroscopically. The savings to the patient are impressive with respect both to physical discomfort and time of recuperation. Considerable financial advantages accrue to the providers of health care. Those procedures most commonly performed include excision of septa, removal of polyps and submucous myomata, endometrial ablation and removal of dense adhesions.

7: Prevention and Management of Complications

No surgery is without risk. Complications of hysteroscopic surgery can occur.

Anaesthesia

The risks to the patient, up to and including death, are no different from those when any general anaesthetic is administered. Prevention rests in ensuring that the patient is in all respects fit enough to withstand a general anaesthetic and in entrusting her care to a skilled anaesthetist. Management will be the responsibility of the anaesthetist who may well recommend that the surgeon immediately discontinue the procedure and return the patient to the supine position.

Positioning the patient

Incorrect or clumsy positioning of the patient may result in:
1 nerve injuries;
2 back injuries;
3 damage to the soft tissue; and
4 deep venous thrombosis (DVT).

Nerve injuries

The degree of Trendelenburg position is always less than that used for operative laparoscopy. Incorrectly placed shoulder restraints or leaving the patient's arm in an extended position on an arm board can result in brachial plexus trauma. Fifteen minutes is all that is required for such a lesion to develop. Prevention rests in the hands of the anaesthetist who must ensure that shoulder restraints and arm boards are used correctly. Replacing shoulder restraints with a non-slip mattress can be very helpful. Pressure on the peroneal nerve from the lithotomy stirrups may result in paraesthesia and foot drop. The surgeon must be satisfied that the legs are correctly positioned.

Should nerve injury occur, consultation should be sought with a neurologist. Fortunately most lesions will resolve spontaneously but recovery may take several months. These injuries are a constant source of delight to malpractice lawyers.

Back injuries

The anaesthetized patient is defenceless against traction injuries to the lumbar spine. Clumsy lifting and lowering of the legs can damage the spinal ligaments resulting in chronic lower back ache. The legs should always be lifted simultaneously by two assistants. They are kept together until they have reached the appropriate height, separated and placed in the stirrups. Removal post-operatively follows a reverse sequence. Little but sympathy and physiotherapy can be offered to a patient who has suffered such an injury.

Damage to the soft tissues

The soft tissues and hands are at risk from the moving parts of the operating table, particularly the hinged or removable foot piece. It is the responsibility of the surgeon to ensure that such accidents never occur. In addition, any metal part of the table and monitoring leads can act as return plates for electrical energy. Burns can occur at these points of contact. The patient must not be touching any metal table parts and all monitoring equipment must be properly insulated.

Deep venous thrombosis

If prolonged pressure is exerted on the calves by lithotomy stirrups, DVT can occur. Ensuring that the lower legs are protected from any pressure is the best prevention. If it is suspected that DVT, or worse, pulmonary embolism has occurred, the advice of a physician (internist) should be sought. If the diagnosis is confirmed anticoagulant therapy will be required.

The distension media

Carbon dioxide is used for diagnostic hysteroscopy. Almost all complex hysteroscopic electrosurgery is performed using either sorbitol or glycine. Saline may be used with the laser. High molecular weight dextran is of value if mechanical dissection with scissors is to be performed. If excessive amounts of the distension media are absorbed the following complications may occur.

Carbon dioxide

- Cardiac arrhythmias.
- Gas embolism and (rarely) death.

Sorbitol

- Hypoglycaemia in the diabetic.
- Haemolysis.
- Fluid overload with acute pulmonary oedema and high output cardiac failure.

Glycine

- Nausea and vertigo.
- Hyponatraemia.
- Fluid overload.
- Transient hypertension followed by hypotension associated with confusion and disorientation.
- Elevated blood ammonia levels leading to encephalopathy, coma and (rarely) death.

Saline

- Fluid overload.

High molecular weight dextran

- Anaphylaxis.
- Adult onset respiratory distress syndrome.
- Pulmonary oedema.

Management will be dependent upon the symptomology.

Carbon dioxide induced cardiac arrythmia or gas embolism will be managed by the anaesthetist.

Hypoglycaemia in diabetic patients is treated by administration of glucose, measurement of blood sugar levels and restoration of euglycaemia.

Haemolysis is rarely of such severity to warrant transfusion. Renal and liver function should be monitored.

Fluid overload predicates insertion of a central venous line, administration of a diuretic, oxygen, and if necessary, cardiac stimulants. A blood pressure cuff may be applied to each limb in rotation to occlude venous return, and in effect perform a bloodless phlebotomy.

Hyponatraemia is treated by the administration of diuretics and hypertonic sodium chloride solution combined with monitoring of the serum electrolyte values until normality has been regained.

Coma and encephalopathy due to elevated blood ammonia levels may require haemodialysis to be performed.

Anaphylaxis is treated by the administration of oxygen, antihistamines, glucocorticoids, and intravenous fluids.

Adult onset respiratory distress syndrome will require the administration of glucocorticoids, oxygen, and occasionally, assisted ventilation.

These complications almost invariably occur in the immediately post-operative period. It is the responsibility of the surgeon and/or anaesthetist to begin immediate resuscitative measures and make the appropriate consultation. Intra-operative occurrence of any of these events warrants immediate cessation of the operation.

Prevention of these complications is achieved by:
- using a distension medium appropriate to the procedure;
- using delivery systems appropriate to the medium;
- keeping fluid pressures below 80 mmHg;
- keeping carbon dioxide pressures below 200 mmHg and flow rate below 100 cm^3/minute;
- keeping operating times to a minimum;
- avoiding entering the vasculature.

If a fluid medium is being used, complications are avoided by:
- maintaining meticulous measurements of fluid intake and output.

• abandoning the procedure if intake exceeds output by more than 2 l or if the anaesthetist encounters signs of early venous congestion.

The surgery

Complications of the specific procedures may occur intra-operatively or be of later onset. Intra-operative complications include the following:

1 failure to complete the procedure;
2 uterine perforation; and
3 haemorrhage.

Late onset complications include:

1 infection;
2 discharge;
3 adhesion formation; and
4 failure of resolution of the presenting symptom.

Intra-operative complications

Failure to complete the procedure

This may occur because it is not possible to visualize the uterine cavity adequately, because complications arise necessitating abandonment, or because the procedure proves to be too difficult.

Management will hinge upon the decision to make a further hysteroscopic attempt at a later date, or to use an alternative approach. The patient must be involved in the decision making. Prevention is achieved by:

• use of appropriate instruments and distension media;
• avoidance of complications;
• proper patient selection.

Uterine perforation

The uterus may be perforated by:

• the dilator;
• the hysteroscope;
• the surgical equipment.

Management will depend upon the severity of the perforation, the means by which it was made, the site of the perforation, the likelihood that an intra-abdominal organ has been damaged, and whether or not laparoscopic monitoring was in progress.

Simple perforations of the fundus can be made with the dilator or hysteroscope. The event should be suspected to have occurred if the dilator passes to a depth greater than the known depth of the uterine cavity. The hysteroscope should always be introduced under direct observation. Learners who pose the question 'what's that' and surgeons who answer 'that's the small bowel' will recognize perforation when it occurs. It is unlikely that an intra-abdominal organ will have been damaged. If the instrument has perforated laterally there is a real risk that a broad ligament haematoma may develop.

Complex perforations are made with scissors, the resectoscope or the laser. It is unusual for scissors to have damaged an internal organ. Internal burns with the resectoscope to any adjacent organ can occur. The laser poses an exceptional hazard. Once the myometrium has been breached it will vaporize the next surface in its path. Even if the bowel has been displaced into the upper abdomen, safety is not guaranteed. If not directly observed, the clue that perforation has occurred will be sudden loss of distension pressure and increase in flow rate.

If perforation is suspected the flow of medium should be stopped and any electrical or laser power switched off immediately. The instrument should be left *in situ*. If laparoscopic monitoring was in progress the severity of the uterine defect can be assessed immediately, and the perforating instrument withdrawn. Any bleeding will be noted. Intra-abdominal structures can be examined to detect any damage. If a broad ligament haematoma has begun to form, its size and rate of growth can be observed.

Damage to an internal organ, severe uterine bleeding, or rapidly growing haematomata warrant immediate repair either by operative laparoscopy or laparotomy.

If the procedure was not monitored laparoscopically the decision must be taken to observe the patient or to intervene actively. It is usually safe to observe patients in whom the perforation was caused by a dilator, the hysteroscope or scissors. The instruments are removed. Active intervention is only indicated if there is severe vaginal bleeding, evidence of a rapidly growing haematoma or of intra-abdominal trauma.

Perforation with electrical current poses a nice clinical dilemma. It is usually better to lean on the side of caution and perform an exploratory laparotomy. This course is mandatory if the laser has been the cause.

Perforation can be prevented by:
• gentle cervical dilatation;

- introduction of the hysteroscope under direct vision and refusal to advance the telescope if the view is obscured;
- using an energy setting appropriate for the procedure;
- making all cutting strokes (where feasible) from the fundus towards the cervix;
- recognizing the thinness of the cornual regions;
- discontinuing dividing a septum as soon as bleeding occurs;
- recognizing the high risk in patients with adhesions or partially intra-mural fibroids;
- obeying the first law of holes which is: 'when you find yourself in a hole stop digging'.

Haemorrhage

Intra- or post-operative bleeding can be caused by:
- the tenaculum;
- the dilators;
- uterine perforation;
- the procedure.

Management will be dependent upon the cause, site and severity of the bleeding.

Cervical laceration caused by the tenaculum or dilators

The final step of any operative procedure is to ensure that such an event has not happened, by reinserting the speculum and visualizing the cervix. Obvious bleeding points can be controlled with pressure from ring forceps or by inserting a figure of eight suture.

Uterine perforation

It is rare for heavy bleeding to follow. If such an event does occur, laparotomy must be performed and the bleeding area oversewn.

Bleeding caused by the procedure

This should be instantly obvious. It may be possible to identify and spot coagulate the vessel involved. If coagulation fails to control the flow the operation is abandoned. A Foley catheter is inserted and the ballon distended. This tamponade can be remarkably successful. The catheter remains *in situ* for 24 hours. Antibiotic cover is given. The presence of the catheter may cause quite severe cramps. Analgesics including prostaglandin synthetase inhibitors may be required.

If these simple measures fail to arrest the haemorrhage a life-saving hysterectomy, or ligation or ultrasound guided embolization of the anterior branches of the internal iliac arteries may be necessary.

The amount of resuscitative measures required, including administration of oxygen, plasma volume expansion and blood transfusion, will be dictated by the amount and speed of blood loss.

Prevention

• The cervix must be dilated gently.
• The surgeon must recognize those steps in any procedure which may predispose to haemorrhage and which include:
   (a) the final incision in dividing a septum;
   (b) resection of embedded fibroids;
   (c) resection which penetrates too deeply into the myometrium if the endometrium is being ablated with the loop rather than the roller ball.
Electrodes should always be in motion when current is being applied. Spot coagulation should be of brief duration.

Late onset complications

Infection

Acute pelvic inflammatory disease is fortunately rare. The diagnosis is made when the classic symptoms and signs become manifest. Management is effected by admission and the administration of fluids, analgesics, the procurement of the appropriate bacteriological (both aerobic and anaerobic) cultures, and the intravenous administration of high doses of antibiotics.

If, as is highly unlikely, a pelvic abscess should develop it will need to be drained.

Prevention

• Correct pre-operative assessment and antibiotic treatment if indicated.
• Avoid any intervention if there is evidence that the patient is suffering from (acute) pelvic inflammatory disease.
• Recognize that those procedures which will result in prolonged passage of necrotic tissue (myomectomy and particularly endometrial ablation) pose a greater risk of infection.

Discharge

If fragments of excised tissue remain in the uterus when a procedure has been completed they will be discharged over the next few days or weeks. This is particularly true in cases of roller ball endometrial ablation. Little can be done to minimize this effect. The patient should be warned to expect the discharge.

Adhesion formation

Any of the complex hysteroscopic surgical procedures which leave raw surfaces may stimulate the formation of intra-uterine adhesions. This is particularly so when dense adhesions are divided or if ablation is performed with the Nd : YAG laser.

Prevention and management

• Where possible, as in the case of fibroids, leaving two raw opposing surfaces should be avoided. It is better to carry out two resections separated by 2 or 3 months.
• Electrosurgical ablation is probably preferable to laser ablation. The former generally leaves an accessible uterine cavity. The latter does not. No long-term studies have been completed in these patients. There is concern that occult carcinoma of the endometrium could arise and remain undetected if there is not free access to the cervix and vagina for the warning symptoms of bleeding.
• An intra-uterine device and adjunctive estrogen and progesterone therapy should be used following resection of adhesions (see Chapter 6).
• Second look diagnostic hysteroscopy may be performed about 6 to 8 weeks post-operatively after complex hysteroscopic surgery. At this time any adhesions will be soft and easily broken down.

Failure of resolution of the presenting symptom

If a surgical procedure does not correct the symptom for which it was performed this can be regarded as a complication. Prevention is based on a combination of:
• proper patient selection;
• meticulous attention to the details of the performance of the surgery.
The scope of this book precludes a detailed discussion of the

outcome of the complex hysteroscopic procedures but a few notes regarding overall failure rates will be made.

• Excision of septa. Approximately 15% of women who conceive will experience a first trimester loss following excision of a septum. The risk of third stage complications is higher in such patients.

• Myomectomy. Insufficient information is available to quote long-term failure rates when myomectomy is performed to control heavy bleeding. In the short term about 20% do not benefit. The outlook is disappointing in infertile patients. Eighty per cent will not conceive.

• Endometrial ablation will fail to ameliorate the symptoms in about 15–20% of patients. If necessary the procedure can be repeated. The long-term sequelae are under active investigation.

• Adhesiolysis in the infertile patient will not be followed by success-ful pregnancy in from 60 to 80%. The prevalence of third stage complications in those who do deliver is high.

• World experience with the treatment of heterotopic bone forma-tion is limited. There is a reasonably high rate of recurrence.

Conclusions

Complications can, and will, arise but can be minimized by careful attention to patient selection and the details of the surgery.

8: Safety and Training

Introduction

Although the first hysteroscopy was performed by Pantaleoni in 1869, the technique has been slow to gain acceptance. Modern diagnostic hysteroscopy has been pursued actively by a small group of enthusiasts since the early 1970s. Laparoscopy did not become widely used until it became apparent that it had a surgical as well as diagnostic role. The same evolution is now occurring with the use of hysteroscopy. Many established gynaecologists who did not have the opportunity to acquire the skills during their training, and junior staff alike, are entering a new field. It is essential that anyone who wishes to learn hysteroscopy understands how maximum safety can be achieved and pursues a course of training in the performance of both diagnostic and operative techniques.

Safety

The preceding chapters have described the indications for, contra-indications to, and complications of diagnostic and operative hysteroscopy. This section will provide a check list of safety procedures.

General

• Procedures should only be carried out by fully trained surgeons or learners under supervision.
• There must be a valid indication.
• There must be no contra-indications.
• Informed consent must have been obtained.

Equipment

Prior to beginning the procedures the surgeon must confirm that:

• all telescopes, sheaths and ancillary instruments are in working order;
• light sources and cables must be functioning and appropriate for the procedure to be performed;
• any electrosurgical generator must be compatible with the electro-surgical instruments and ground electrode;
• all insulation must be intact and the working parts of the electro-surgical instruments fully functional;
• lasers should be calibrated and performing perfectly;
• distension media should only be delivered by an appropriate insufflator (in the case of carbon dioxide) or pump (in the case of non-viscous fluids). Recommended pressure and flow rates should not be exceeded;
• the medium used should be appropriate to the procedure to be performed.

The procedures

• The patient's general state of health should not preclude the use of general anaesthesia.
• The patient's general state of health should not place her at risk should fluid overload occur.
• Local anaesthesia should be administered initially as a small test dose to identify any patient who might suffer an allergic or idiosyn-cratic reaction.
• During diagnostic hysteroscopy the telescope should not be ad-vanced if all that can be seen is a red circle. This may represent blood on the lens or the uterine wall.
• Operative procedures should not begin until the surgeon is satis-fied that the landmarks (usually the tubal ostia) have been identified.
• Particular care must be taken with the use of electrosurgery or laser energy at the tubo-cornual junction.
• The use of intra-operative ultrasound can reduce the risk of uterine perforation during operative procedures.
• When fluid media are used during prolonged surgeries, strict attention must be paid to the intake and output.
• Patients should be observed for several hours post-operatively to ensure that signs of fluid overload, or encephalopathy if glycine has been used, will be detected early and can be dealt with.
• Certain procedures, that is those where the teacher cannot see what the learner is doing, can be a source of great anxiety. This can be greatly diminished if a silicone chip camera is used during all instructional sessions.

If these steps are followed meticulously, complications should be rare indeed. The first prerequisite was that the surgeon be fully trained. The next section will address the issue of training.

The fundamentals of training

1 Assessment of departmental needs.
2 Provision of facilities.
3 The learning process.

Assessment of departmental needs

The needs of the department will depend upon:
   (a) the need to provide service;
   (b) teaching;
   (c) research.
It may be judged appropriate to concentrate some procedures in the hands of a limited number of individuals. These matters should be discussed and agreed upon by the members of a department before the period of formal training begins.

Facilities

Provision of the necessary equipment and operating room time for the performance of any procedure may limit the number of individuals to be trained. It is important that those who are trained can begin to work in their parent institution immediately upon completion of their training.

The learning process

The learner should be a qualified gynaecologist or registered gynaecologist in training. A series of steps should be undertaken and include:
   (a) acquisition of the knowledge;
   (b) learning and performing diagnostic hysteroscopy;
   (c) learning and performing hysteroscopic surgical procedures of increasing complexity.

Knowledge

Several excellent texts are available. Many didactic courses are offered internationally. The pupil must understand:

- the instruments;
- the principles of electrosurgery;
- the principles of laser surgery;
- the indications, contra-indications and risks;
- the management of complications;
- the techniques of diagnostic hysteroscopy;
- the appearances of the hysteroscopically identifiable lesions;
- the techniques of operative hysteroscopy.

Diagnostic hysteroscopy

There are two steps:
- acquisition of the basic skills;
- practice.

The basic skills can be acquired by attendance at a well-run basic 'hands on' course or by working with a skilled colleague. A series of exercises can then be carried out in the surgeon's own unit:

- Examination of hysterectomy specimens. Once the uterus has been removed, the tubes can be clamped, hysteroscopy performed and the uterus divided so that the surgeon can compare any lesion observed hysteroscopically with its actual appearance. This approach can be humbling. Often apparently massive lesions will be seen to be small indeed.

- Performance in the anaesthetized patient. The first attempts at hysteroscopy must be under general anaesthesia when there is time to practice on a suitable subject. The most favourable patient is the parous woman of childbearing age with a normal sized uterus of less than 8 cm in length.

Once the surgeon is confident that the basic skills have been mastered, the final step is to begin to use the carbon dioxide hysteroscope in an out-patient setting. The first few cases are best performed using local anaesthesia.

Out-patient hysteroscopy should not be attempted until successful procedures to instill confidence in the surgeon have been performed under general anaesthesia. It is important not to be in too great a hurry. Time spent in familiarizing oneself with the instrument and its assembly, learning the extent and, particularly, the direction, of the field of vision when an oblique lens is used, and on the choice and properties of the distension medium will be amply repaid by the speed with which the trainee's expertise increases. While most hysteroscopists favour carbon dioxide as the distension medium for diagnostic hysteroscopy, it may present problems for the beginner. Bleeding provoked by the hysteroscope negotiating the cervical canal usually prevents further examination and bubbles produced by the cervical mucus may also make visualization difficult. The learner will often find it easier to use a fluid medium such as 32% dextran-70 in 10% dextrose (Hyskon) before progressing to carbon dioxide hysteroscopy.

Having become a competent diagnostic hysteroscopist the gynaecologist is ready to begin learning hysteroscopic surgery.

Surgical hysteroscopy

The would-be surgical hysteroscopist must undergo:
1 changes in attitude;
2 acquisition of knowledge;
3 formal training; and
4 practice.

Changes in attitude. The majority of gynaecologists have been primarily trained in abdominal or vaginal surgery and, possibly later in their careers, have developed an interest in laparoscopy and hysteroscopy. When commencing operative hysteroscopy the surgeon must appreciate that the instruments are different from those used in conventional surgery and it may frequently be difficult for senior surgeons to adapt to these new techniques, and to accept that they must acquire new skills. Indeed the more experienced they are in the old operations, the more difficult it may be to change to new ones and the learning curve may therefore be significantly longer than for a younger, more adaptable person.

The surgeon must learn to operate in a new environment and accommodate to the two-dimensional image offered by the telescope, and then learn to operate off the video screen. This latter technique should be adopted as soon as possible in the training period as in many cases it is difficult to work without it. In addition to learning to use the new instruments, the surgeon must appreciate their capabilities, their risks and their limitations. Initially the staff in the operating room must accept that operations may take longer although, with experience, hysteroscopic surgery will take approximately the same or even less time than conventional surgery. Most experienced surgeons should be able to complete endometrial resection or ablation in an average of 20–40 minutes. The nursing staff must also learn to use the new instruments in order to function as a team. This will be helped by the use of video cameras so that they can see the operation and, when necessary, assist in its performance.

Acquisition of knowledge. The surgeon's knowledge base as described earlier should be re-enforced by reading and attendance at didactic sessions.

Formal training can be acquired:
- at courses or in a colleague's unit;
- in the surgeon's parent institution.

Before undertaking operative hysteroscopy, the surgeon must have extensive experience in diagnostic hysteroscopy. At all times a clear view of the uterine cavity must be obtained. The surgeon must know to stop the operation if vision is compromised. Tragedies have resulted from inexperienced hysteroscopic surgeons failing to appreciate this when the uterine distension system has failed, and continuing to use high frequency current or laser, resulting in perforation of the uterus and damage to organs such as major vessels, ureter and bowel. There can be no fixed rule for the number of diagnostic hysteroscopies which one should perform before proceeding to operative hysteroscopy as everybody's learning curve is different and, in recent years, the teaching of endoscopy has improved to such an extent that any arbitrary number is meaningless.

Courses. Initially the gynaecologist may obtain an overview of the possibilities by attending conferences where hysteroscopy is discussed or, better, where live operations are relayed to the auditorium from the operating room. Video recordings make excellent teaching aids but they can be criticized because editing can make the operation look easier and better than it really was. Few surgeons will produce a recorded video containing the failures of their techniques as well as the successes.

Conferences are organized in many countries in Europe and North America, either sponsored by institutions, or by the instrument manufacturers to whom much credit must be given for the interest in education and safety promotion in these techniques. National and international societies are now developing in many countries which seek to educate by means of endoscopy courses, and to monitor the success of the procedures and the incidence of complications. Their meetings also provide a forum for discussion and allow the surgeon who wishes to learn operative hysteroscopy to listen and watch the expert at work.

Courses using a workshop format should last 1–2 days and include lectures and discussion on the theory and practice of hysteroscopy. The groups should be small enough to allow all the participants to contribute and to have the opportunity of 'hands on' training. Six surgeons is probably the ideal number, and in order to obtain the maximum benefit from the workshop they should already have some preliminary experience in diagnostic hysteroscopy and have attended at least one larger conference. Longer attachment to a training unit is desirable but not always possible because of financial constraints and the time involved. There may be inefficient use of time if the trainer has limited access to the operating room and so a week at a centre may only allow attendance at two or three operating sessions.

Initial training can commence on an inert model consisting of a plastic case, with a replaceable wax lining resembling the uterine cavity which can be excised by the resectoscope loop without using electricity. Biological tissue can be provided by an excised bovine uterus, which is larger than the human organ but provides a readily available substitute on which to practice the use of the instruments. Alternatively an excised human uterus can be used *in vitro* to gain experience before commencing hysteroscopic surgery.

In organizing a workshop, practical experience should be offered in diagnostic hysteroscopy initially under general anaesthesia and then in an out-patient setting before proceeding to operative hysteroscopy. If they are sufficiently experienced, each trainee can be allowed to perform part of the operation, treating some of the uterine cavity with the resectoscope or laser under close supervision using the video screen. Attending such a course is strongly recommended before seeking attachment to a colleague.

When the surgeon has gained experience in diagnostic hysteroscopy and has attended courses, conferences or workshops where the scope, risks and complications of operative hysteroscopy will have been learnt, further benefit can accrue from attending a colleague's operating session and learning on a one-to-one basis.

Having demonstrated general ability the trainee can be allowed to perform more operations under supervision than are possible at a workshop; the development of surgical skills will probably increase faster and with greater safety than if the learner were to work unsupervised.

At the surgeon's parent institution. Some units have been remarkably successful at arranging in-house training. A great degree of co-operation between surgeons and the operating room staff is required. Usually a week is scheduled so that the didactic part of the course, taught by the visiting expert/s precedes 3 or 4 full days of 'hands on' instruction in the operating rooms.

Practice. The final step is practice. As with any newly acquired skill it is sensible to move from the simple to the complex. Chapters 5 and 6 have discussed the simple and the complex operative procedures.

The gynaecologist should become thoroughly comfortable with performance of the simple before attempting the complex. It is recommended that as the learner progresses from simple to more complex procedures, each step of increasing difficulty should be mastered under the supervision of a recognized expert. As with diagnostic hysteroscopy it is helpful to begin with patients who are anaesthetized before transferring these skills to the out-patient department.

This mastering of the simple procedures will take time. If the learner feels that the time is of such duration that the techniques of major hysteroscopic surgery learnt at the training course have become rusty, a refresher course or several sessions spent working with a skilled colleague are recommended before embarking on such procedures unsupervised.

It is recommended that division of dense adhesions, resection of septa, resection of fibroids and endometrial ablation be performed initially under laparoscopic control. While this approach will not prevent uterine perforation it can ensure that if such an event were to occur the bowel could have been removed from contact with the uterus and thus is not at risk. The severity of damage can be assessed immediately.

Conclusions

Diagnostic and operative hysteroscopy are valuable, safe procedures provided that:
1 safety precautions are meticulously observed; and
2 training has been logical, thorough, and effective.

Index

Italic numerals refer to illustrations.